AF775845

Precious Pills

Series: Epistemologies of Healing

General Editors: David Parkin and Elisabeth Hsu, Institute of Social and Cultural Anthropology, Oxford

This series in medical anthropology will publish monographs and collected essays on indigenous (so-called traditional) medical knowledge and practice, alternative and complementary medicine, and ethnobiological studies that relate to health and illness. The emphasis of the series is on the way indigenous epistemologies inform healing, against a background of comparison with other practices, and in recognition of the fluidity between them.

Volume 1
Conjuring Hope: Magic and Healing in Contemporary Russia
Galina Lindquist

Volume 2
Precious Pills: Medicine and Social Change among Tibetan Refugees in India
Audrey Prost

Precious Pills

Medicine and Social Change among Tibetan Refugees in India

Audrey Prost

First published in 2008 by

Berghahn Books
www.berghahnbooks.com

© 2008 Audrey Prost

All rights reserved. Except for the quotation of short passages for the purposes of criticism and review, no part of this book may be reproduced in any form or by any means, electronic or mechanical, including photocopying, recording, or any information storage and retrieval system now known or to be invented, without written permission of the publisher.

Library of Congress Cataloging-in-Publication Data

Prost, Audrey, 1977-
Precious pills : medicine and social change among Tibetan refugees in India / Audrey Prost.
p. cm. -- (Epistemologies of healing ; v. 2)
Includes bibliographical references and index.
ISBN 978-1-84545-457-9 (hardback : alk. paper)
1. Medical anthropology--India. 2. Medical anthropology--Tibet. 3. Traditional medicine--India. 4. Traditional medicine--Tibet. 5. Tibetans--Medicine--India. 6. Tibetans--India--Social conditions. 7. Refugees--Tibet. 8. Refugees--India. I. Title.

GN296.5.I4P76 2008
306.4'610954--dc22

2008014702

British Library Cataloguing in Publication Data

A catalogue record for this book is available from the British Library

Printed in the United States on acid-free paper.

ISBN: 978-1-84545-457-9 (hardback)

For my family

Contents

List of Figures and Tables

Figures

Tables

Acknowledgements

I would like to express my deepest gratitude to the many people who helped me during fieldwork in Dharamsala. Dr Dawa (Mentsikhang), the late Dr Tenzin Choedak, Dr Dickyi Tsomo, and Dr Tseten offered help and insights. For their support and humour, I wish to thank friends Tenzin Lhawang, Jamyang Tenzin, Tsering Tendel, Tenzin Tsultrim, and Lobsang Gyatso at the Library of Tibetan Works and Archives. I am grateful to Norzum and her family for looking after me during the first half of my stay. Humble thanks are also due to Tashi Tsering of the Amnye Machen Institute for his insightful research suggestions, to Sangye Tendar Naga for his teachings, and to Nyima Phuntsok's family for their kind support. I have not named friends and informants who contributed stories of illness, but my biggest debt is obviously to them. Alexandra Correia, Paula Sharp, Stuart Yeh, Frédéric Geri, Sanna Allsopp, Claire Colomb, Nathalie Rivère de Carles, and Murielle Cozette offered friendship and inspiration. Dr Yoshitaka Ota and Dr Etsuko Ota were generous beyond all expectations.

I am also grateful to the various persons who have read and offered suggestions on drafts of this work: my supervisors Dr. Mukulika Banerjee and Prof. Murray Last, Prof. Phil Burnham and Prof. Danny Miller at University College London, Dr. Martin Mills and Dr Martin Potter, as well as to my thesis examiners, Dr. Charles Ramble and Prof. Geoffrey Samuel. Prof. Murray Last provided much inspiration as well as some of the photographs included in this book. I am particularly indebted to Barbara Gerke from Oxford and the International Trust for Traditional Medicine, and to Dr Mona Schrempf at the Humboldt Universität zu Berlin for their invaluable comments and advice. The shortcomings of this work are, however, entirely my own. This book is dedicated to the students of Dharamsala's Mentsikhang, who serve patients with insight and compassion despite the traumas of exile.

Note on Transliteration and the Wylie System

Many of the quotes inserted in this book are translated from the Tibetan. Others are from interviews in which English was the main language used. English-language interviews are marked with an asterisk (*). In the interest of clarity, phonetic spelling is used for Tibetan terms in the main text and in tables. Wylie spellings can be found in the glossary at the end of the book, along with a list of key historical figures and places. Some Tibetan extracts from interviews can be found in notes at the end of each chapter. I have used Wylie spelling for these and initial capitalisation at the beginning of sentences.

The terms 'refugee' and 'exile' are used interchangeably in this book, since Tibetans refer to themselves as both. India is not a signatory of the 1951 United Nations Refugee Convention and Tibetans therefore do not have official refugee status in India. Tibetans who arrived in India before 1980 have a right to permanent Indian residency.[1] Tibetans who arrived after 1980, on the other hand, are given a residence permit which they must renew every year. Newly arrived Tibetans do not enjoy the full rights of Indian citizenship (they cannot vote or carry an Indian passport), but they are free to work and own property in India. In practice, Tibetans describe themselves either as refugees or as exiles, and I have therefore used both terms throughout the book.

Notes

1. In the form of 'RCs' (Residential Certificates), which allow Tibetans to work and have domestic travel rights, and 'ICs' (Indian Identity Certificates), with which Tibetans can travel abroad.

List of Abbreviations

BCG	Bacillus Calmette–Guérin, used in vaccination against tuberculosis
CMO	chief medical officer
CTA	Central Tibetan Administration
DOTS	Directly Observed Treatment (Short Course)
HP	Himachal Pradesh
MBBS	Bachelor of Medicine, Bachelor of Surgery
MTK	Mentsikhang (Dharamsala)
PRC	People's Republic of China
RCT	Randomised Controlled Trial
TAR	Tibet Autonomous Region
TB	Tuberculosis
TCHRD	Tibetan Centre for Human Rights and Democracy
TCV	Tibetan Children's Village
UNHCR	United Nations High Commission for Refugees

Introduction

This book is about the production of 'public health' in the context of displacement. Through an ethnography of the social and medical worlds of a community of Tibetan refugees in India, I examine the following questions: how does long-term displacement affect concepts of health, and how are traditional medical systems modified through the needs of displaced populations?

What does it mean to speak of the 'production' of public health? Public health is concerned with the protection and improvement of population health through community effort, preventive medicine and research. An inclusive definition of public health therefore encompasses biomedical interventions but also social and political interventions (Anand et al., 2004).

Why is an anthropological study useful to understand the production of public health? Population scientists, epidemiologists and anthropologists have devised a number of tools with which to assess the health of populations. Many of these approaches seek to pinpoint a discretely measurable 'health status' defined by macro-level markers such as morbidity, birth, death, and fertility rates, or the distribution of acute and chronic diseases. While indicators such as household income or employment status provide useful information, the standardisation produced by rigid categories of data often glosses over sociocultural factors critical to understanding conceptions of health at a local level. Bourgeois refers to statistical inconsistencies as the 'dirty linen' of epidemiology, and argues that 'rather than exploring intellectually the meanings of the limits of their datasets, [epidemiologists] instead dismiss, ignore, or subject excessive rounds of "multivariate control" onto statistically significant associations between behaviours and outcomes that are counterintuitive or embarrassing' (Bourgeois, 2002: 260). It is hard to 'control' for social life: even after carefully constructing categories of socio-economic status, finding just what aspects of socio-economic position affect health remains a difficult task. Although 'cultural' and 'social' epidemiologists have taken up this challenge (Braveman et al., 2005; Trostle and Sommerfeld, 1996; Trostle, 2005), others prefer to keep social life – including socio-economic status – as a 'black box'.

The use of anthropological theory and methods may help to redress this disengagement with the sociocultural factors that influence health. Anthropologists involved in ethnographic work on health and well-being tend to focus on small-scale communities, distinct groups, or individuals. This gives anthropology a different vantage point to other health sciences like epidemiology or demography, which are largely concerned with determinants of health and illness at a population level. Ethnographic accounts enable researchers to see how well-being and ill health are produced in everyday life by examining the social processes behind health-seeking behaviour (the practical things that people do in order to maintain or return to health), as well as the content and organization of local medical practices (what is done about health complaints and how these are interpreted in local medical discourses). A long tradition of ethnographic studies has demonstrated that traditional medicine plays an important role in maintaining well-being by addressing key social concerns related to health and providing locally appropriate responses to illness. Ethnographic research can also document the social strategies through which communities address and remedy ill health. Recent anthropological studies, for example, have explored how small-scale communities cope with violence or displacement, and shown how individual and social well-being is 'recovered' through ritual, political, and everyday social practices (Valentine, 1996; Das et al., 2001; Argenti-Pillen, 2003). This study is premised on the widely accepted notion that anthropology can contribute to public health research by bringing social and cultural practices to bear upon questions of health.

This book offers two main arguments. The first is that displacement affects the health of communities differentially: in the Tibetan case, socio-economic inequalities internal to the diaspora influence the health status of individuals negatively; thus, not all refugees are equal when it comes to health. While much research has focused on ill health within the broad context of host–migrant relationships (Ahearn, 2000; Grove and Zwi, 2005), little is known about the ways in which social inequalities internal to particular diaspora groups combine with external ones to influence health. Furthermore, what little we know comes from studies of health inequalities within diasporas in Europe and the USA, and there have been few studies of health inequalities within 'South–South diasporas'. Drawing upon data collected during thirteen months of ethnographic research among Tibetan refugees in India, this book illustrates some of the ways in which socio-economic disparities within diasporic communities impact on health status and health-seeking behaviour.

The second argument put forward by this book is that traditional medical systems can be seen as public health resources because they articulate key social concerns about health and provide culturally meaningful answers to them. Moreover, far from being fixed bodies of knowledge, traditional medical practices are influenced by political and social changes, and thereby come to reflect societal changes. The next two sections examine each of these claims in more detail.

Socio-economic inequalities and health among diaspora communities

In recent years, renewed attention has been given to ways in which displacement affects the health of diaspora populations (Aspinall, 2001; Nazroo, 2001). Epidemiological studies, in particular, have demonstrated that social inequalities are linked to ill health (Wilkinson, 1996; Graham, 2002; Pearce and Smith, 2003; Marmot, 2004). This research has implications for understanding health within diaspora communities: anthropological studies show that diaspora groups are heterogeneous, that inequalities exist within them, and that these inequalities, in turn, impact upon health. Anthropologist Aiwah Ong gives a striking example of this. She describes the way in which personal and kinship bonds (*guanxi*) are called upon to strengthen business networks across the Chinese diaspora in South-East Asia (Ong, 1999). But while *guanxi* is 'enabling' because it strengthens trade networks, it also effectively keeps women and the poor 'out of business' and is 'basically a structure of limits and inequality for the many and of flexibility and mobility for the few' (Ong, 1999: 117). Diaspora networks and the values that sustain them may be enabling, but they can also be constraining. Indeed, some of them may generate social inequalities that have negative impacts on health (Fadiman, 1997; Gardner, 2002; Nguyen and Peschard, 2003). This book addresses the issue of social inequality in the context of the Tibetan diaspora in India; in particular, it examines why some refugees are more at risk of illness than others.

What can traditional medicine tell us about the health of migrants?

Epidemiologists and anthropologists have shown that migrants often face an increased risk of morbidity and mortality compared with non-migrants (Aspinall, 2001; Nazroo, 2001; McKay et al., 2003). However, the links between migration, environmental factors and disease are not straightforward. Their interaction is mediated by factors related to socio-economic status and social support. The way that these factors combine and contribute to the increased burden of morbidity among migrants, however, is poorly understood. In the case of the Tibetan exile community in India, the absence of accurate longitudinal and cross-sectional data makes it difficult to carry out 'traditional' epidemiological studies. Demographic data collected in 1998 show that Tibetans constitute the largest refugee group in India, with a population of over 118,000 scattered over thirty-six large settlements and Indian urban centres (Central Tibetan Administration, 2000). Health surveys conducted in the settlements demonstrate that the community is slowly undergoing an epidemiological transition: it is shifting away from a morbidity and mortality burden primarily caused by communicable diseases like TB and malaria, to a burden of disease characterised by non-communicable conditions such as cancer and diabetes (Bhatia et al., 2002a; Punkhill, 1992). Data gained from 'verbal autopsies' indicate that cancer, tuberculosis, accidents, cirrhosis, and heart disease are the main causes of death in Tibetan refugee communities (Bhatia et al., 2002a). These data are patchy, however, and, while they offer some measure of disease in the Tibetan community, they tell us little about whether, and how, migration has impacted on health.

A number of studies in exile Tibetan communities have looked at the mental health consequences of displacement. Mental health specialists working with Tibetan exiles have reported high levels of depression and post-traumatic stress disorder among newly arrived Tibetan refugees (Crescenzi et al., 2002: 374). However, many studies also highlight the positive contribution of Buddhist spirituality in coping with depression and anxiety.[1] In fact, most studies on Tibetan refugee communities emphasise the role of culturally specific practices and knowledge systems – such as Buddhist practices – in coping with displacement.

Few studies, on the other hand, have looked at the role of traditional medicine in Tibetan exile communities. This oversight should be corrected for a number of reasons. First, traditional Tibetan physicians are present in all exile settlements, and traditional clinics are widely used health-care facilities. Secondly, traditional Tibetan medicine is given political support by the Tibetan government in exile, and traditional physicians play a critical role in promoting healthy behaviour in exile settlements. Thirdly, traditional Tibetan medicine addresses health problems in the context of Buddhist spirituality and culturally constructed views of the body. Studying the contemporary use of Tibetan medicine can therefore help us to understand how Tibetans deal with displacement within their own 'emic' understandings of illness and treatment.

In this ethnography, I argue that traditional Tibetan medicine provides culturally meaningful ways of dealing with the somatic and psychological consequences of displacement. I report results from a small survey of prevalent diseases in Dharamsala (see Chapter 3), showing that many exiles relate diseases to environmental and moral changes specific to exile. These form the core of chronic exile discomforts that Tibetan medicine is particularly apt at dealing with. The book also shows how long-term displacement acts as a catalyst for change in local concepts of health and illness, and is dialectically implicated in the transformation of traditional Tibetan medicine. It attempts to demonstrate that traditional Tibetan medical practitioners, far from being simply 'reactive' to social change, actively contribute to changing local concepts of health.

Central to this work is an idea put forward by Leslie (1976): traditional medical systems are by no means static entities, but rather social, political, and economic forces in their own right. This book also contends that traditional medical systems can be viewed as a public health resource, not because traditional doctors can or should be employed for biomedically informed health promotion, but because their medical practice allows them to tap into emic understandings of disease and react swiftly to the health implications of social change.

Methodology and ethical concerns

Data for this book were gathered during thirteen months of fieldwork in Dharamsala (Himachal Pradesh, India). They include: (1) questionnaire-based data on prevalent diseases and their causes, which were collected among seventy-four attendees at a biomedical and a traditional Tibetan medical institution in Dharamsala (the Mentsikhang); (2) participant observation data from both institutions gathered over the course of six months each; (3) thirty-two in-depth interviews with patients in both institutions; (4) data from thirteen months of participant observation with Tibetan refugees and their families in Dharamsala.[2]

During the first period of fieldwork, from October 2000 to September 2001, I remained in the middle settlement of Gangchen Kyishong (henceforth Gangkyi). During a second stay from June to July 2002, I lived in a group of flats shared by Tibetans in the Library of Tibetan Works and Archives in Gangkyi. My first four months in Dharamsala were spent on intense language training with an instructor in McLeod Ganj. I then established contact with the two most prominent health-care providers in Dharamsala. The first, known as Mentsikhang, is a provider of traditional Tibetan medicine. The second, Delek Hospital, is a biomedical facility. At the Mentsikhang, I learned medical vocabulary and elements of clinical medicine. I interviewed twelve traditional doctors on their daily practice. Eight of these physicians were from Mentsikhang, and four others had trained there and set up independent clinics.[3] I also interviewed fifteen students at different stages of the Institute's curriculum. In Delek Hospital, I volunteered on the TB ward and accompanied friends on their visits to relatives on the ward. I interviewed five nurses and four volunteer members of staff. My involvement with these two prominent medical institutions naturally raised the issue of informants' protection. I have changed the names of all practitioners and patients in this book, and asked for patients' consent to use the information given by them through the questionnaires and interviews.

Researching Dharamsala

Contemporary studies of Tibetan exiles have, until very recently, suffered from a bias against Dharamsala (Diehl, 2002; Klieger, 2002). After the publication of the town's first household census in 1984 (Saklani, 1984), the majority of research on Tibetans in India focused on documenting life in rural exile communities, such as the settlements of Darjeeling and Kalimpong (Subba, 1990), or Mundgod in Karnataka (Palakshappa, 1978). In the literature as well as among Tibetologists, there was a sense that, like post-1950 Tibet, Dharamsala embodied the gradual demise of traditional Tibetan society. Exile life was seen as an atrophied vestige of its former Tibetan self. Scholars and visitors unofficially derided it as an adulterated field of anthropological enquiry, 'inauthentic' and little worthy of investigation. Friends and students at university usually referred to my research site as belonging to a broader Tibetan cultural whole ('so, when you were in Tibet'), or depicted it as a hot spot on the Indian spiritual tourist circuit ('where did you go again, Rishikesh?').

Defining authenticity is a local matter before and after it becomes an anthropological 'problem': Tibetan exiles themselves question the authenticity of Dharamsala as 'little Lhasa in India'. One anthropologist accurately describes this unease: 'Dharamsala displays a deeply ironic landscape, in that its claim to Tibetan legitimacy exists among scores of tourist souvenir shops, hotels, chai huts, and cake and donut restaurants, none of which ever existed in traditional

Tibetan cities … yet Dharamsala is a place where memories and nostalgia for a lost way of life are perpetuated as no other.'[4]

Many early studies of Dharamsala were premised on the assumption that Tibetan exile identity was only worth studying in so far as it contained traces of 'how things were in the past' (in Tibet), and how well exiles could retain these features. In these 'adaptation studies', anthropologists unequivocally agreed that Tibetans had been extremely successful in retaining their ancestral way of life in the face of acculturation, and were a model of good integration with their host populations (Fürer-Haimendorf, 1990; Palakshappa, 1978; Saklani, 1984; Subba, 1990). Little was said, however, about what exactly these 'endangered traditions' might have been, or what conflicts had arisen in the process of preserving them.

In recent years, the substantial growth of publications on and by Tibetan refugees has reversed this tendency to essentialise exiles as 'Tibetans by proxy' (Alam, 2000; Diehl, 2002; Ardley, 2003). As Chinese influence in the Tibet Autonomous Region continues to grow (Ramble and Buffetrille, 1998), Tibetan refugees in India are increasingly construed by Western audiences as the only true representatives of Tibetan culture. This view is informed by the widely held belief that Buddhism is the dominant marker of Tibetan identity; in the Western imagination, it then often follows that 'true' Tibetans are those who are able to express their religious beliefs and to participate in the preservation of a Tibetan culture devoid of Chinese influences.

This more recent portrayal of Tibetan exiles is a product of Tibet's ambigious relationship with the West. Tibetans have long been 'prisoners of Shangri-La', a Western myth that construed Tibet as a remote and mysterious land, and described Tibetans as quintessentially religious and devoid of materialistic preocuppations (Lopez, 1998). Contemporary accounts of Dharamsala perpetuate the fantasy of Shangri-La:[5] few televised documentaries about the town show anything more than its main Buddhist temple, prayer gatherings, and celebrations for the Dalai Lama's birthday. While such events have deep significance in the context of exile, these local meanings often elude the viewer. Instead, the overall effect is to reinforce the stereotype of Tibetans as religious zealots, and to further entrench the myth of Shangri-la. A more sensitive portrayal of Dharamsala is given by the Indian writer Pankaj Mishra:

> Something of the private and incommunicable melancholy of permanent exile hung over its huddled houses and perched streets … ageing men with broad, lined faces sat still and pensive behind jars of sticky sweets. They looked remote and abstracted even while talking to you, and you wondered what memories of lost homelands were decaying behind the piercing sadness of their stoic faces.[6]

The melancholic Tibetan dreaming of 'lost homelands' can indeed be found in Dharamsala's dusty roadside tea-shops. Next to him, however, and incongruous with Dharamsala's 'little Lhasa' image, are young second-generation Tibetan refugees bartering in Hindi, newly arrived Tibetans watching Chinese action films and chattering monks filing outside internet cafes.

Dharamsala is heritage-conscious, yet also evolving at a spectacular pace. It is possibly the most cosmopolitan Tibetan community in India, comprising Tibetans from across traditional Tibetan cultural areas, and from widely diverse social backgrounds. It is a regional trade hub and has considerable exposure to foreigners through tourism.[7] The town is now part of the Himalayan 'hippie trail', and is linked through trade and business networks to other neighbouring ex-'hill stations' (e.g. Simla and Manali), the greater Himalayan tourist circuit (including Ladakh and Nepal), and key sites of spiritual interest (e.g., Rishikesh, Varanasi and Bodh Gaya). Because of its key role as seat of the Tibetan government in exile, educational centre, and trading hub, Dharamsala is also at the heart of migration networks. Its population is highly mobile: traders come to Dharamsala from other Tibetan settlements to sell their products, and students return home to Dharamsala from their neighbouring campuses. Monks and nuns from Dharamsala travel to receive Buddhist teachings, while others come from South India to sojourn in Dharamsala's highly esteemed monasteries.

Western influence is increasingly felt in Dharamsala. The Tibetan cause's considerable exposure to world attention has had deep repercussions on the small exile community. Dharamsala is highly dependent on foreign aid and tourism, and this has strongly contributed to the rise of Western influence in the town. For many Tibetans and foreigners in Dharamsala, modernity is presented as an exchange in which both parties have prescribed roles: Tibetans share with visitors the rich spiritual heritage of Buddhism and, in return, are offered sponsorship for children's education, money for biomedical clinics and for institutions preserving the 'traditions' of Tibetan culture. Underpinning this exchange is a tacit contract that encourages exiles to retain their culture in order to deserve the aid they receive (Prost, 2006b).

Previous studies of Tibetan communities have tended to adopt a unilaterally damning approach to social change, indicting any loss of tradition as a sign of growing cultural anomie. In early studies of exile communities, social scientists were primarily interested in measuring the Tibetans' progression towards acculturation and assimilation as part of a generalisable 'experience of exile'. Yet several social scientists have rejected such a focus on 'adaptation' and 'uprooting' because it presupposes that refugee communities are homogeneous and respond to the pressures of exile in a uniform manner (Malkki 1992, 1995a, 1995b; Morrissey, 1983). Tibetan refugees come from a broad range of social and economic backgrounds, and this very fact undermines the possibility of writing the history of a common, homogeneous 'acculturation'. Indeed, recent studies have highlighted Dharamsala's distinctiveness as the product of nearly fifty years of exile (Diehl, 2002).

I question the relevance of research agendas that try to chart the Tibetans' awareness of their 'roots' and heritage. The dangers of acculturation are certainly on people's minds: they are endlessly discussed in public speeches and gatherings where Tibetan youths are exhorted by older refugees to 'remain Tibetan'. Nevertheless, the 'uprooted' have grown roots. The community of Dharamsala already has a history of its own: three generations of exiles have built their lives in the small hill settlement. Many young Tibetans speak of a distinctly 'Dharamsala' culture, with its own idiomatic language, local community networks, and a style of being and acting recognisable among other Tibetan exile communities.[8] Indeed, research on Tibetan identity in the diaspora describes the strong cultural self-consciousness that characterises exile cultural productions (De Voe, 1983; Harris, 1999).

This book participates in the recent research effort to uncover Tibetan exile modernities (Diehl, 2002; Klieger, 2002). It seeks to chart some of the social changes affecting Tibetans in Dharamsala and further afield by examining local concepts of health and changes in the practice of traditional medicine. The book is divided into two main sections. Part I addresses the issue of social inequalities in exile, and looks at the impact of socio-economic differences between more established Tibetans and newcomers in relation to health and health-seeking behaviour. Part II is given over to an investigation of the role of traditional Tibetan medicine in sustaining public health in exile, and looks at recent changes in the theory and practice of traditional Tibetan medicine.

Notes

1. Holtz, 1998; Crescenzi et al., 2002; Mercer et al., 2005.
2. The response to the questionnaire was only partially satisfactory as far as information about health was concerned, but provided a good starting point for discussing family histories. Part of the limitation of the questionnaire lay in the fact that few Tibetans spoke openly about serious medical conditions. The tendency to gloss over subjective appraisals of illness is a commonly reported problem with the use of questionnaires and structured interviews in both anthropological and epidemiological studies.
3. Two of the non-Mentsikhang doctors were reluctant to have their account inserted in the study, and I have therefore omitted them.
4. Klieger, 2002: 3.
5. With the exception of Diehl's (2002) account of music in the Tibetan exile community.
6. Mishra, 2000: 218–19.
7. One particularly aggressive local shop-owner was referred to as '*bilkul nyonpa*' (literally, completely crazy) by young Tibetans in my area. Such expressions mixing Hindi and Tibetan were commonly used by children of the Tibetan Children's Village (TCV) and referred to as 'TCV-speak'.
8. Studies of exile culture have come under criticism for being exclusively focused on Dharamsala, and for reifying a 'story' of exile primarily constructed by Tibetan administrators, intellectuals, lamas, and 'cultural performers' who are conversant with, and eager to engage in, debates

about Tibetan culture on terms set by Western audiences, as Toni Huber (1999) argues:

> In my own experience, most Tibetan refugees are not like these persons, and certainly do not live in Dharamsala, but in rather non-cosmopolitan agricultural and craft communities. They tend to be humble and self-effacing, conservative, often uncritically devoted to their leaders, seemingly as avid about watching Hindi films as attending religious ceremonies, and they have Hindi or Nepali, not English, as their second language. Why are these many Tibetan exiles left backstage or merely out in the audience in the study of 'Tibetan culture?'

Part I
Inequalities in Exile

Chapter 1
'Because we are Tibetans ...': Talking about Health

This chapter introduces Dharamsala through four fieldwork episodes that focus on individual Tibetans' experiences of health problems in exile. The data for these case studies were recorded in 2000 and 2001. The aim of this chapter is to provide ethnographic contextualisation for the issues further developed in this book.

Health warnings at the theatre

Every year, a springtime theatre competition is held in Dharamsala, home to the largest community of Tibetans in India. Most of the plays deal with local issues, and many echo dominant concerns in the Tibetan exile community: the struggle for Tibetan independence, foreign support for a free Tibet, and Dharamsala's salient health problems.

This year's final act opens onto a stage resembling the local hospital's tuberculosis (TB) clinic. Two beds face the audience. In the first, an emaciated young Tibetan boy breathes the characteristic wheeze of tuberculosis, coughing out bloodstained sputum. In the second bed, a rotund diabetic Tibetan elder grumbles over the measly portions of hospital food, and attempts to bribe relatives for sweets and alcohol.

The tuberculosis patient tells the audience and his ailing room-mate the story of his escape from Tibet. Risking death just to find oneself in a crowded camp in India with no employment prospect, and now afflicted with tuberculosis, 'Why carry on?' he asks the audience. 'Rather die,' he adds, with youthful bravado. The young newcomer hides his medication under the pillow without taking it. Nurses fail to notice that he has stopped taking the pills and regularly sneaks out to the balcony to smoke cigarettes given to him by his diabetic roommate. The pair decide on a strategy to fool the hospital personnel: the diabetic patient smuggles in cigarettes through his visiting wife and daughter, which the tuberculosis patient exchanges for his share of food and sweets.

In this truculent scene, a Tibetan newcomer and an 'old-timer' (a first-generation refugee) bond despite the social differences that had previously kept them apart. Soon enough, however, their trickery is exposed. The nurses find a stack of untouched pills under the young TB patient's pillow. It is already too late: in a dramatic flourish, the young man rises from his bed, his face mask tainted with blood, and collapses on stage. Meanwhile, the diabetic elder, who has been feasting on rich foods and Tibetan butter tea, gives in to a great convulsion and falls dead into the arms of his weeping wife and daughter. In the audience, the commotion and laughter caused by the two men's performance descend into an uneasy silence.

Onstage comes the biomedical doctor, a real-life civil servant. The make-believe doctor makes the following pronouncement:

> Because we are Tibetans, we are kind to each other, we help each other. But if we do not listen to the doctors, if we do not listen to the nurses, we are putting each other in danger. If we all get sick here, if our children die here, how will we go back to Tibet? If you want to truly help each other, be vigilant to disease.

Offstage, I contemplate the truthful depiction contained in this play: newcomers and 'old-timers' do find each other on opposite sides of the epidemiological transition. While newcomers suffer a disproportionate burden of communicable diseases such as TB, 'old-timers' are also at risk but more often bear the brunt of chronic illnesses (Nelson et al., 2001). Clearly some of this is age-related; however, age does not explain everything. The socio-economic conditions which newcomers find themselves in upon arrival in India may be telling the other half of the story. What has barely begun to emerge in the local hospital's data sets is already popular knowledge among local Tibetans: newcomers, exposed to poor living conditions and poverty, are at risk for diseases like TB. The vulnerability of newcomers was to be confirmed some time later during a visit to the local biomedical hospital.

A night at Delek Hospital

A few months after the play, I sit on the balcony of Delek Hospital, at the top of the real-life tuberculosis clinic. Patients next to me survey the passers-by. Night falls and the conversation is scarce. What needs to be said by way of introduction has been said a long time ago. Now conversations are mostly about bodily needs, fatigue, and foreseeable visits from relatives.

Shortly after midnight, a young man is brought in by ambulance, struck down by a drug overdose. The nurses tell me he is a newcomer, a newly arrived Tibetan refugee. The boy passes away around four o'clock in the morning. Monks from the nearby monastery promptly arrive at the hospital with a bagful of ritual implements: bells (*drilbu*), drums (*damaru*), and the Tibetan book of the dead (*bardo thodol*) strapped in its orange cloth. The monks perform the first rituals of the bardo in the hospital, chanting over the young man's covered face. The other patients look on, their faces sombre with apprehension.

Outside the room where the monks sit, a nurse explains that many of the emergencies in the hospital are drug-related: young newcomers driven to despair by the lack of opportunities in exile take to drugs as a consolation. Two Tibetan boys staying on the ward comment that other newcomers will arrive from Tibet before the New Year (*losar*) in February: many Tibetans undertake the risky passage across the border to Nepal to be reunited with family for the great prayer festival (*monlam*) in Dharamsala. This means that there will be more patients in the hospital. Many newcomers fall ill during the journey, or in the crowded refugee reception centre in Dharamsala. Some, like the young man who passed away that night, will die of drug abuse and despair. He is the first of many to come, the boys tell me.

The morning after this incident, the ward is buzzing with activity: the outpatients TB clinic starts and patients huddle in the corridors with relatives and friends. However, for those staying on the TB ward, time stretches on.

Namgyal, a 23-year-old India-born Tibetan refugee, reflects on his condition after two months of treatment on first line TB drugs: 'I have no body strength', he starts. Then, almost as a corrective afterthought, he adds: 'Inside my body, there is no strength. I cannot walk out of this room you see. So the world is my room. My brother came to visit yesterday; he also had TB [*TB natsa*] two years ago. Now he is better.' He adjusts himself on the bed, pulling up his legs and propping his back against the wall.

> I often think this medicine is making my body sick. But I don't know about this disease, I don't know the cause [*kyen*] of it. Yes, I know the cause is ... a bu, bacteria, but why are you not sick? [He laughs and pulls out his tongue.] You have the BCG, and Tibetan children get it too, but they still get sick. Maybe there is a special problem with Tibetans and with Indians. With these new diseases, like TB, it's like there is a war inside your body.[1] When I see old people with TB, I feel I am not the only one who experiences suffering [*dugnyel*]. Old people have a virtuous mind [*sem dewa*]; they really use the mind as a guide, to understand the disease. I am not so good. Usually, I am confused.[2]

'Why are you not ill?' Namgyal knows exactly why, but he is too polite to say. He eats a single meal of rice and dhal a day, and lives in a small room with a leaky roof, which he shares with five other young Tibetan men. Two of them have had TB already. Namgyal's story is typical of many newcomers: after coming out of the 'transit' school where young newcomers are usually accommodated after arriving in India, he worked as a waiter in a cafe that provided 'sustainable employment' for Tibetans. Namgyal served organic carrot cake to well-meaning tourists for six months, but 'sustainability' stopped when the tourist season ended. He then sold Tibetan dumplings by the roadside in pilgrimage sites for ten rupees a bag (approximately twenty cents). He lived in tents and rented rooms with other Tibetans: traders, sweater-sellers, and monks. In the summer of 2000, Namgyal returned to Dharamsala for the Dalai Lama's annual teachings. Then the first symptoms of TB arrived. When I interviewed him, Namgyal was undergoing treatment on the tuberculosis ward, and wondered what would happen to him after leaving the hospital. In 2002, he went back to Tibet.

But many newcomers simply cannot return to the TAR, or they would risk being caught and sent to prison. During my first months in Dharamsala, I often sat in the pharmacy of the traditional medical clinic (Mentsikhang) and observed newcomers receiving their prescriptions. One of them was Lhamo. The story that follows unfolded after one of her consultations at Mentsikhang.

Lhamo's consultation

Lhamo, a recently married 32-year-old Tibetan woman, arrives at the Mentsikhang complaining of abdominal pain. Her Tibetan doctor is a young female practitioner. She takes out the registered notebook in which she has written Lhamo's old prescription, and asks if she has been taking her medicines regularly. Lhamo nods, and says: 'Yes, Shiru in the morning then Agar 20 in the evening with hot water, one precious pill [*rinchen mangjor chenmo*] on the full moon day, and golden needle [*ser kab*] treatment once every two months.' Lhamo adds quietly: 'I have done everything except the golden needle, but I would like to try now.'[3] 'I thought it would be dangerous, but now I think it is worth trying,' she adds.

'Allright,' says the doctor, 'come and take a seat.' Lhamo sits down facing the doctor and puts her left arm forward. Using her right hand, the doctor places three fingers on Lhamo's left wrist and adjusts her fingers on each radial artery, almost imperceptibly counting the pulsations under her breath. She then proceeds to examine each radial artery's pulse individually with both hands. The entire exercise lasts about ten minutes. Her occasional explanations concern the particular organs she is sensing through her fingers. The doctor says she is particularly concerned about Lhamo's *samseou*, an organ associated with reproduction and menstruation. 'This pulse is "sunken" [*ching*], and it is the middle of the month.' 'This is a difficult case [*sokai ne*]', she says. 'You haven't had your period [*da tsen*] this month, have you?' she asks. 'No,' Lhamo replies, 'not for four months now ... I had some bleeding last August, but it was only two days, and it looked like "old blood" [*nying thrag*], it was not red.' 'Have you been eating nuts, milk and many cold foods?' the doctor asks. 'I have been drinking some milk. I have tried to eat more meat, but it is expensive.' The doctor replies:

> That is good, you must eat, you must strengthen your body. Eat meat but not much, otherwise you will feel tired and sleepy. You can eat fish and mutton. Eat foods with strong, hot [*tsa*] and sharp [*no*] taste during the first half of the month, and you must stop taking the precious pill at that time. We will not do the golden needle treatment just now, we will wait until the spring. I will give you some medicine to treat your phlegm, but we must be careful not to increase your wind humour [*lung*], so do not do too much exercise or work too hard.

Lhamo smiles and I sense an unspoken understanding between the two women. Perhaps my presence is making them uncomfortable.

Upon her arrival in India, Lhamo joined the 'sister nunnery' of her home institution to continue her studies. She then met a young local Tibetan man and decided to marry. However, Lhamo feared the consequences of 'disrobing' (leaving the nunnery) and felt she would miss the camaraderie of other nuns. In fact, her old friends from the nunnery were never very far, as I soon noticed, and came to visit whenever they had a chance. Many of them had suffered at the hands of the Chinese, and Lhamo herself had been locked up in the nunnery for two months before escaping to India.

One day, as I sat with them having tea, Lhamo's husband Pasang said they wanted to have children. They had been trying for some time without success, and this was what had prompted Lhamo's visit to the Mentsikhang. Lhamo's husband said his wife was not strong and needed to eat more. Lhamo, on the other hand, thought it was a bad idea to disrobe after being a nun for so long, and that this was causing her present difficulties. I asked another female doctor from the Mentsikhang how being a nun could affect one's health:

> Being a nun is very good, because you gain a lot of merit. But changing can sometimes be difficult because your body is not used to intercourse with a man, because when you are a nun, even if you are old, you are like a virgin [*mosar*]. So some elements are not strong in your body. To make a child you need two things. First, the child comes through the karma [*le*] of parents, this brings the wind humour [*lung*] into the womb [*ngel*]. Then, at a certain time, the substances [*kuwa*] of man and woman must come together. For the woman, she must have enough red element [*kam marpo*] in her seminal vesicle [*samseou*]

to make a child. If the red element does not arise, then you cannot have a child. There can be many other problems after that too, but this is the main problem for nuns. So first you need to treat phlegm [*beygen*], which is cool and like water, so that the red element can arise.

I then understood Lhamo's predicament. She was well versed in religious practice and fearful of the negative consequences of leaving the nunnery. However, she trusted the young Mentsikhang doctor treating her: 'the doctors [at Mentsikhang] have deep compassion, they understand the suffering of people here. They are good to nuns who have been tortured or raped. They understand, they speak to them kindly.'

When I returned to Dharamsala in 2002, Lhamo and her husband were expecting their first child. Lhamo had never visited the biomedical hospital. As I saw them sitting together, I did not have the heart to ask what treatment she had used, and what rationale lay behind it. But I did ask if she was enjoying her new life. She said:

> Everything changes ... one minute you are sitting, relaxing with your friends, laughing and eating good food, the next you are alone, poor, with nobody to talk to, your parents have passed away ... That is why you take refuge in the three jewels [the Buddha, the dharma and the sangha], because they are unchanging. Now I have this child, this husband, this house, but tomorrow maybe the Indians will not want us here anymore. Everything changes. Now I am a housewife, but it may change.

Her husband glanced at us. 'This one is still very religious,' he said lovingly. I tried to think of one of the witty Tibetan proverbs that Lhamo had taught me as a repartee, but my memory failed, and so I nodded. She went to the kitchen to fetch our lunch, and, as I followed her in, I noticed the brand new rice cooker on the concrete workspace. When I congratulated her on their new purchase, Lhamo pouted in feigned disappointment: 'It is Chinese,' she said in an apologetic tone, and exploded with laughter. Who were the traditional practitioners who helped treat patients like Lhamo?

In the course of my stay, I developed a relationship with one of them, a young physician by the name of Thagpa. Over the course of several months, Thagpa revealed his journey as a practitioner of traditional Tibetan medicine.

Thagpa: the makings of a traditional Tibetan doctor

In 2000, Thagpa was a 30-year-old medical student at the Mentsikhang, Dharamsala's traditional Tibetan medicine institute. The middle child of three, he was born in a family of farmers from the eastern outskirts of Lhasa. When the time came for him to decide where to continue his studies after secondary education, Thagpa told his parents about his plan to take the entrance examinations for the Mentsikhang in Dharamsala. They disapproved. After much reflection, Thagpa left the house without saying goodbye to his parents, and set out on the journey to India via Nepal. Thagpa recalled how, just before leaving Tibet, he had a dream vision of the Dalai Lama sitting on a white horse, waving to him and urging him to come forward. He viewed this as an auspicious omen for the journey.

Soon after crossing the border into Nepal, Thagpa and his travelling companion were arrested by a border patrol. The Nepalese soldier took their identity papers and threatened to take them back to the border if they did not give him money. Thagpa and his friend gave up the savings they had brought along for the trip. Hungry and frightened, they found help in a Buddhist monastery, and finally made their way to Kathmandu, where they received new papers and some money for the fare to India. Shortly after his arrival in Dharamsala, Thagpa joined the transit school for newcomers in Bir, where he stayed for three years learning Hindi and English.

During his time in the rough tin barracks of the Tibetan transit school, Thagpa contracted pulmonary TB. He was sent to Dharamsala's biomedical Delek Hospital for treatment. The school was a breeding ground for disease: students lived in barracks of fifty, and, with few showers and toilets, hygiene was poor. Thagpa recalled the humming monsoons in the transit school, and students driven to desperation by the hammering noise of rain on the tin roofs, unable to concentrate, unable to go out. He had already lost five kilos by the time he was admitted to Delek Hospital. Thagpa's general health was poor: like many young Tibetans in Lhasa, he was a heavy smoker (he referred to himself as a *dogong*, or chimney), and had a penchant for fatty Tibetan dumplings. The Western doctors who worked as volunteers at Delek Hospital knew Thagpa was taking Tibetan medicine alongside his biomedical regimen, and encouraged him to continue this combination. Thagpa explained that western doctors had told him Tibetan medicine 'could do no harm' because it was 'like vitamins'. With treatment, his condition improved dramatically. Thagpa was finally discharged from the hospital after two months of continuous TB treatment, and took drugs under the supervision of a health worker for another four months.

Three years after this episode, Thagpa joked that cigarettes had saved him from TB, but then, correcting himself, said that his karma (the consequences of his actions in past lifetimes) had led him to be cured. Thagpa's experience had not dented his motivation to study Tibetan medicine: quite the contrary. He successfully sat the examination for entry into the Mentsikhang's five-year astrology course. His command of Tibetan grammar and writing skills was much appreciated by his fellow students, and he rapidly became a respected member of the student body.

I saw Thagpa regularly throughout the winter of 2000, and, after some time talking to him about his studies, our conversations turned to the topic of his family and life in Tibet. Unlike most recent refugees I had spoken to, he was quite reluctant to discuss these issues. Thagpa had not spoken to his parents since his departure, and only occasionally sent and received news through a woman he called his 'aunt' (*ani*), in reality a distant cousin who lived in McLeod Ganj. When I met him, he had not written to his parents for a year. He dreaded telling them about starting another five-year course at Mentsikhang to become a doctor, after which he would find work in one of the institute's branches as a traditional Tibetan physician (*menpa*). He felt embarrassed about being a student at the age of thirty, and about not being able to support his parents.

In the years that followed his recovery from TB and his entry into the Mentsikhang, Thagpa said that he often suffered from a sad mind (*sem gyopo*), irritability (*lung tsapo* or 'hot wind'), as well as from stomach and skin disorders. He blamed these on an increase of the wind humour (*lung*), since *lung* is often implicated in changes in mental states. He also diagnosed himself with a great susceptibility to *beygen* (phlegm) imbalance. This was in turn linked to his *lung* disorder (lung is thought to guide the general humoral behaviour of the body, and therefore aggravate *beygen* conditions). This predicament, he diagnosed expertly, was further exacerbated by the hot and cold transitions of the Indian climate, changes to which he remained highly sensitive even after nine years in exile.

Thagpa thought that his increase in *lung* had triggered episodes of low mood, which were worsened by guilt about leaving his family, and doubts about his abilities as a student. He also felt guilty about his unusually high consumption of alcohol and cigarettes. This particular problem caused Thagpa much angst: he worried that his professors and fellow students would see him drinking in the restaurants of Lower Dharamsala. These bars and pool rooms were the domain of second-generation Tibetan exiles, a group looked down upon by more conservative Tibetans as unruly.

During episodes of low mood, Thagpa went for *mo* divinations (dice divinations performed by monks or lay practitioners). His preferred *mopa* was a famous practitioner who lived in the nearby old people's home in Dharamsala. In the spring of 2001, the *mopa* advised Thagpa to take refuge in the Buddha Maitreya, and encouraged him to go to the Dalai Lama's annual teachings. According to the *mopa*, the underlying force behind Thagpa's frequent mood disturbances was undoubtedly *le ngen*, negative karma. Thagpa attended the teachings and took repeated vows to stop smoking and continue his spiritual practice. When he failed to uphold the vows, he complained of irrepressible headaches (*go ne*), of a lazy mind that prevented him from learning his texts by heart (*katon du she me pa*), and of 'athlete's foot' (in his own words). This last condition signalled that, as he put it to friends one evening, everything in him, even his feet, had started to 'rot' (*rulwa*).

Thagpa's *mopa* felt that the medical therapies for these problems would only work in combination with a strengthening of ethical discipline, more recitations, and more spiritual practice. Thagpa persevered, and his experiences of illness and hardships reinforced his motivation to become a doctor: he saw in the medical profession a form of redemptive existence, a way to ameliorate his karma. Thagpa graduated from the Mentsikhang in 2002 after ten years of study. He now practises traditional Tibetan medicine in one of the most remote

Tibetan settlements in Ladakh (north India), a place that is, in his own nostalgic words, 'much like Tibet'.

Tseyang: a neighbourhood tackles tuberculosis

A few months after my arrival in Dharamsala, TB struck again in a family close to me. Ani Tseyang-la, a 62-year-old nun, had fallen ill after one of her room-mates from the nunnery had contracted the disease. Tseyang had a 43-year-old son, Norbu, as well as relatives living in other local Tibetan settlements. She had decided to become a nun after the death of her husband and her son's marriage. Norbu's wife, her daughter-in-law, had left Dharamsala to live in Canada, from where she sent money home to her husband. The family's main sources of income were the money coming from Canada and Norbu's salary as a low-paid assistant in one of Gangkyi's institutions. Tseyang experienced her first TB symptoms during the winter of 2000:

> I am really not well. First, I got breathing pains. I started to cough everyday, no blood, just coughing and sometimes it was so much, I had nausea. One of my friends, a nun, had just been sick with TB. I had helped her go down to the hospital, take her medicine, and sometimes brought her food when she was down [in the hospital]. I had a mask when I helped her but sometimes I took it off. You cannot speak clearly with the mask, and you cannot recite mantras.

During the winter, Tseyang left the nunnery to come and stay with Norbu in his two-bedroom flat in a quiet part of McLeod Ganj. There she attempted to recover from what she thought might be a *lung* imbalance, or perhaps, she said, *gulcham*, a 'cold throat'. Norbu hardly ever left his mothers' side: 'even if he wants to go somewhere, he doesn't dare,' their neighbour Rinchen told me.

Norbu and Tseyang visited a local lama twice for *mo* divinations at the onset of her illness. After a few weeks of hearing Tseyang's prolonged coughing, Norbu became convinced that she had tuberculosis. He even put an ear to her back and chest to try to detect the wheezing sound or 'crackles' that doctors listened for with their stethoscopes. Tseyang continues: 'Norbu took me to the hospital for the first time when he heard me cough. I wanted to have a divination [*mo*] to find out if I would die soon. I am old, am I not? I thought it was a good time, the right time.' The doctors at the hospital immediately diagnosed pulmonary tuberculosis.

After the diagnosis, Tseyang increased the frequency of her religious recitations in preparation for the time when the biomedical therapy would stop sustaining her pulse, which she felt was an indicator of her strength. She knew that TB was not necessarily fatal but thought she was too old to survive it. Her apprehension grew when she learnt how long the biomedical treatment would last. Norbu claimed she wanted to die, that she thought she was beyond treatment, and deliberatly tried to avoid taking her biomedical drugs, though she would not stop taking Tibetan medicine.

A great number of people became involved in Tseyang's care. Norbu accompanied Tseyang to her weekly appointments with the Tibetan TB specialist who examined her X-rays and delivered the prescriptions. Norbu's neighbour and friend, a non-practising nurse, offered to administer Tseyang's daily injections so that she would not have to stay in the hospital or constantly travel up and down the hill for treatment. Meanwhile, Tseyang swallowed some of the *mani rilbu* brought back by her family from the temple. She could now no longer walk safely down the road to the hospital alone. Her family thought that TB (*tibi natsa*), caused by the bacteria of TB (*tibi sin bu*), was weakening her, causing her body's strength (*luki nupa*) to diminish. A friend of Tseyang, also a nun at nearby Gaden Choeling, said that she could see her life force (*tsesog*) was being used up. Family members were taking turns to bring Tseyang down by taxi on the winding road to Delek Hospital, and I was then called upon to help support her along the painful trip.

After the technicians in the laboratory had taken an X-ray of Tseyang's chest, Norbu and I waited with her on the bench outside the TB specialist's office. We sat in silence, looking at patients and nurses going out of the sickrooms with bedpans and trays of food. Tseyang looked around anxiously, and Norbu held a handkerchief over his mouth. I found the relative anonymity afforded by the mask comforting (as I suspect they did too). Although she was considered a 'compliant' patient and did not openly oppose the trips, Tseyang stayed quietly in a corner, and wore her protective mask and robe over her head so that she would not be recognised. These small acts betrayed her obvious discomfort in the clinic.

At home, she would lie on the family's carpeted bed, resting and reciting *mani*. She usually sat up and reached for the mask lodged under her chin whenever somebody came into the room. Neighbours brought cooked food and helped with the house laundry. On the whole, Norbu carried out most of the household chores and worried about his mother constantly. He felt the strain of his combined duties sharply. Concerns with his mother's health added to his preoccupations with job security, and this in turn contributed to aggravating his drinking habit and a penchant for gambling.

After three months of treatment, Tseyang appeared to be on the mend. Norbu was still taking her regularly to the *mopa*, a local lama. The monk would give them appraisals of the treatment's progress and suggest spiritual practices focusing on white Tara *namgyalma* (known as the 'all-victorious'), and recitations of the Medicine Buddha mantra. Tseyang would recite the mantras before taking her Tibetan medicine and at other times during the day.

One day I came in as Tseyang's neighbour Rinchen, who occasionally moonlighted as a nurse, prepared her TB medicine injections in the adjacent room. Rinchen's present occupation barely allowed her to support her family, and she constantly reported difficulties with her landlord, a Tibetan female 'nouveau riche' (*nordag*, a wealthy person), who was constantly increasing her tenants' rent with, as she described it, no concern for people, no compassion (*nyingje mena*). Although she was not part of the contingent of trained health workers from Delek Hospital, Rinchen helped monitor Tseyang's treatment. I asked her how one could help TB patients.

> These TB patients, when they stay by themselves the whole day, they worry about their sickness… They cannot get better that way. And they don't get tasty food, good quality food, only dhal, rice, potato, bread. TB patients … what do they need? They need a high-protein diet. I know, I worked in a big hospital. Not down here [Delek Hospital], there is a better place. TB patients really need to eat [according to] a special diet, they need to eat vegetables, and meat, and lots of protein.*

Norbu interjects: 'TB is very strong,' but Rinchen carries on:

> Where there is a lot of TB, you have to give lots of talks. Do they have a lot of talks? Nurses, or what is it … social workers, every week, there should be talks, on what to do, how we can prevent it. Prevention is better than cure, the doctors all told us that. Once you get sick then there is a problem. If you are good doctor, if you are a good nurse, you don't think just about your salary!*

She frowns:

> These people [TB patients] they really need help. I have seen some nurses who were really not good. When checking a patient, they would do something like this [She makes the gesture of slapping medicines on a table].
>
> No … When we were training, we worked in the hospital, [we learnt] we must stand near the patient's bedside until he takes the medicine and we should talk, we should give them hope. [Then, affecting a nurse's mannerism] 'You should be happy that you are here in hospital now, we are here to take care of you and you are going to get well with this medicine.' Sometimes these nurses just said: 'here is medicine, take, eat! EAT!' Because [they have] no time … Maybe the patient won't eat the medicine, hide it under the bed. Sometimes patients really suffer, and they worry, and [they] think, 'Taking medicine every day, why?'*

I then question Rinchen about the length of her training as a nurse and whether she thinks people helping their relatives with TB treatment should have specific training.

> If people need help, I help. But 'Yes, yes, I'm a nurse,' I don't say that. For example, [Norbu's] mother, she's very weak, she can't walk. Every week she needs to go to the hospital. Up, down [the hill]. So I said: ask the doctor if he can give us injection [materials] for a week. So they ask Dr. Tseten, he's the highest [in rank] in the TB clinic. From now on, on Monday[s], we will go and take the medicine. Now [Tseyang] it is better, but she is very weak all the time. Until she's better she has to [take treatment]. That's why people get sick, young ones, boys, girls, they take medicine for a while, then they feel better so they don't care. And then they go out till late, they go to parties, dancing, without eating well. OK, if you go to a party, fine, then sleep. Many young people get ill. My opinion is, it is because they don't sleep in time, they don't eat in time, they don't get a proper diet. They think [posturing] 'Oh, I'm getting fat, I can't be fashionable, I should not get fatter.' And then, [you] have to get injections, so?*

Rinchen fixes her apron and steps out onto the common landing, the non-disposable syringes placed on a hospital-like metal tray, ready to give Tseyang her injections.

Through the stories of Tseyang, Lhamo, and Thagpa, we begin to understand some of the ways in which Tibetan exiles experience ill health. Young newcomers often encounter considerable hardship upon migration, and are common victims of infectious diseases such as TB. Older refugees also experience ill health, but are able to draw upon kin networks for support. In the following chapter, I further introduce the Tibetan exile community of Dharamsala, and look at some of the demographic and socio-economic factors behind inequalities in health within the community.

Notes

1. *'Dmar nang bzhin red: nga'i gzugs po nang la rgya gar gyi 'bu a ni chyi gyel gyi sman dmar rgyag res rgyab gyi 'dug'.*
2. *'So sor gyi na tsha'i sems kyi 'dren brtag gyi red [...] nam rgyun la mgo nyog po dug.'*
3. During golden needle treatment, a thin pointed needle is inserted at specific points on the patient's cranium; this is said to be particularly effective in the treatment of *lung* (wind humour) disorders.

Chapter 2
'India is the Happiest Place!': Contextualising Exile

Tibetans: the world's sympathy stock.
Serene monks and bubbly traditionalists;
one lakh [100,000] and several thousand odd,
nicely mixed, steeped
in various assimilating cultural hegemonies.

At every check-post and office,
I am an 'Indian-Tibetan'.
My Registration Certificate,
I renew every year, with a *salaam*.
A foreigner born in India.
(Tenzin Tsundue, *My Tibetanness*, 2005)

Crossing the border

Over 118,000 Tibetans live outside the Tibet Autonomous Region (People's Republic of China).[1] Tibetan refugees first entered India in 1959, after the Chinese invasion of Tibet forced the Dalai Lama to escape across the Indian border. Approximately 85,000 Tibetans followed in exodus (Shakya, 1999). With the support of India's government and foreign aid agencies, Tibetans built temporary government facilities in the small Himalayan town of Dharamsala. The settlement further expanded during the 1960s, when the Sino-Indian border dispute (1962) caused the displacement of recently arrived Tibetan refugees from the frontier areas into the Indian hinterland. More Tibetans then entered India and Nepal during the 1980s, as China temporarily relaxed its hard-line policy in the Tibetan Autonomous

Region and reopened the Tibetan border with Nepal. Finally, following a clampdown on Tibetan immigration at the Nepali – Tibetan border in 1995, the number of Tibetan refugees entering Nepal and India dropped significantly. The United Nations High Commission for Refugees (UNHCR) estimates that as many as 25,000 Tibetans sought refuge in India between 1986 and 1996, and that approximately 1,000 Tibetans continue to cross the border into Nepal every year. There are now thirty-six Tibetan settlements in India.

Recent exile Tibetan surveys show that the population is expanding through natural demographic dynamics as well as through the influx of newcomers from Tibet (Central Tibetan Administration, 2000). The thirteen Tibetan settlements of Himachal Pradesh, where I carried out fieldwork, are home to over 20,000 Tibetans. The Tibetan exile population in India consists mostly of two groups: younger Tibetans (between fifteen and twenty-five years old) and those over the age of sixty-five. Most of the refugees born in Tibet came from the original migration in the early 1960s. A transition therefore occurs in the thirty to 39-year-old age group: only 2.7% of refugees under the age of thirty were born in Tibet. The majority of Tibetan refugees who arrived in India between 1991 and 1996 were between fourteen and twenty-five years old. Many of them were seeking education: 44% were monks and nuns, and 30% were children who joined Tibetan exile schools (Moynihan, 1997). As many as 80% of these new refugees were from the regions of Kham and Amdo, parts of which have been incorporated into the Chinese provinces of Qinghai, Gansu, Sichuan and Yunnan.

While Tibetans will commonly say that escaping religious persecution is their main reason for coming into exile, this may often mask complex stories of economic deprivation, loss, and lack of opportunity in the Tibetan Autonomous Region. Very often, the decision to leave the TAR or Chinese counties is reached through the joint pressure of low socio-economic status and political repression (the 'push' factors), and the promise of employment, further education, or migration opportunities in exile (the 'pull' factors).

Tibetan refugees mainly work in agriculture, trade, and tourism. According to the Central Tibetan Administration, 13% of the Tibetan population in India is involved in handicraft production, mostly carpet weaving. Handicrafts are also a secondary source of income for many Tibetans, and 29% of the population is involved in sweater-selling and clothes trading. Another 30% are employed in services, either in the government or private businesses such as hotels. Dharamsala's population is mostly employed in public services (the government sector) and private business, and by Tibetan standards therefore constitutes a rather elite segment of the refugee community. Although the 1998 census reports low unemployment in the settlement, many exile Tibetans are employed part-time, or on salaries that barely enable them to meet the costs of daily life. Many families are living on the edge of poverty despite being reported as employed (Central Tibetan Administration, 2000).

Dharamsala

The town of Dharamsala encompasses three communities. In the lower part of town is the largely Indian village of Lower Dharamsala, home to a population of Hindus, Muslims, and Sikhs. The main commercial centre, Kotwali Bazaar, is located in this segment of town. To Tibetans, Lower Dharamsala functions primarily as a shopping centre and local transport hub. Indians and Tibetans mingle in the market, but few Tibetans actually live in Lower Dharamsala itself. The population of Lower Dharamsala is largely Indian (*c.* 20,000 inhabitants). Dharamsala is the district headquarters of Kangra and hosts important judiciary and commercial facilities. Inhabitants of Kangra's smaller towns have long relied on migrant work for sustenance and therefore spend several months of the year away in towns like Dharamsala (Parry, 1979). The district courts of Dharamsala, based in Kaccheri, employ a large number of Lower Dharamsala's inhabitants. While the main languages spoken are Hindi, Punjabi, Pahari, and English, many Lower Dharamsala inhabitants involved in commerce have also acquired a basic knowledge of Tibetan.

Halfway up the hill lies the semi-residential hamlet of Gangchen Kyishong, which harbours most of the Tibetan governmental departments and cultural institutions (see Figure 2.1), as well as the biomedical hospital's two buildings. A considerable proportion of

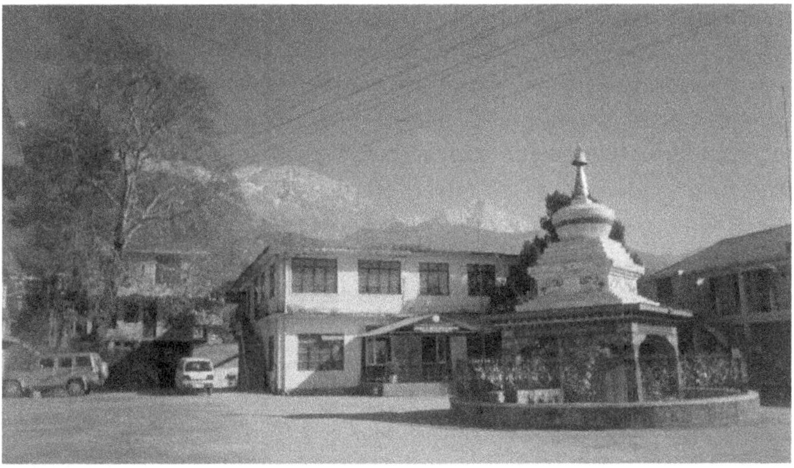

Figure 2.1: Gankyi's main square with the Assembly of Tibetan Peoples' Deputies and the Dhauladhar range in the background. (Photo: Audrey Prost, 2001)

Gangkyi residents are civil servants and work in the different offices of the Central Tibetan Administration. The status of Dharamsala as the 'capital' of the Tibetan diaspora community in India and throughout the world stems from the political and symbolic weight of the CTA, as well as the Dalai Lama's presence in the hill station.

The upper settlement of McLeod Ganj has the largest Tibetan population in India (approximately 9,500 inhabitants) and is rapidly expanding across the surrounding pine forests. McLeod accommodates booming touristic and commercial activities run by both Tibetan and Indian business owners. There are a number of Tibetan and Kashmiri-owned shops, hotels, and restaurants. Dharamsala also houses the town's main Buddhist temple and the Dalai Lama's residence. All three settlements comprised in the greater unit of Dharamsala make up a mixed population of around 29,000 inhabitants.

Since the Tibetans' arrival in Dharamsala in the 1960s, the relationship between Hindu, Muslim, and Buddhist communities has been in a state of precarious equilibrium. In 1972, Saklani conducted interviews in Indian households around the Tibetan settlements of Mussoorie and Dharamsala, and reported that a large majority of her informants were 'critical of the cultural closedness of Tibetan refugees'. They wanted Tibetans to integrate with Indians as much as possible, for example by learning Indian languages and intermarrying with the local population (Saklani, 1984: 380). In 2000, an elderly local Indian shop-owner and ardent supporter of the Dalai Lama explained to me that, in the late 1960s, local people did not think that the Tibetan community would come to play such an important part in the town's life. 'Before the Dalai Lama came here, there was nobody in McLeod Ganj,' he said. 'No cars, no restaurants, no tourists.' Since then, the town had obviously been transfigured.

The growing success of Tibetan businesses has created tension between local Indians and Tibetans. In 1998, a rioting crowd of local Pahari and Kashmiri men raided McLeod Ganj, throwing stones at local Tibetan shops and looting the contents of Tibetan-owned jewellery and handicrafts boutiques. Tibetan shop-owners in McLeod interviewed in 2001 asserted that the raids were carried out with a view to clamping down on Tibetan businesses and incapacitating shop-owners by collecting extortionate fines. This was seen as a mark of discrimination and resentment against the commercial success of Tibetan ventures. The resentment caused by the prosperity of some Tibetan families and businesses has been noted by previous studies (Anand, 2002: 18). De Voe writes that 'jealousy of Tibetan entrepreneurship and benefits bestowed upon them by aid agencies added to their [Indians'] ambivalence about having Tibetans as neighbours' (1983: 20). The label 'refugee' has done some disservice to established Tibetans in Dharamsala. Many now find themselves confronted with the prejudice that they should remain, as one Tibetan Children's Village teacher remarked, 'in rags because we are refugees' (Prost, 2006b).

In reality, however, the wealth generated by Tibetan businesses is concentrated in the hands of a few families in Dharamsala, and much of the population is dependent on jobs that pay very little. Opportunities range from salaried employment in the Tibetan government's many offices in Gangkyi, to teaching or handicrafts work. Furthermore, Tibetans have considerable difficulty in buying land and setting up businesses. The majority of the population earns far less 8,000 Rupees (roughly 200 US dollars) per month, which makes buying houses or flats very difficult for the majority of the

Tibetan population. According to the CTA, only 16.5 per cent of the exile population live in owned accommodation.[2] The costs of buying and maintaining a house in Dharamsala make it hard for a great majority of the population to own their own homes.

In February 2001, I recorded a discussion between a group of young newcomers and an elderly first-generation refugee on this issue:

> **Elderly man:** There are not a lot of wealthy people here. Business people are wealthy, but people like me are not. I live [here] because I can stay in the old people's home and His Holiness [the Dalai Lama] gives me money.
> **Young male newcomer (twenty-five):** We thought we were going to become wealthy here, or at least get some education so we could earn more money in Tibet.
> **Young female newcomer:** You see, this is a mistake. We have nothing here, so how can you expect to make any money? The only money here comes from foreigners, it is *rogram* [sponsorship].
> **Young woman (twenty-four)** [to me, in English]: In my view, we Tibetans are very good business people, but everyone thinks we are just monks and nuns, so they are shocked when we get *rogram* or start our own business because they think, oh ... Tibetans do not care about material things, that we are only, you know, spiritual. But how can you feed your family by just being spiritual?*
> **Young female newcomer:** Yes, and there are a lot of Tibetans doing well in business. But because we are refugees we are not allowed to do as much as we could.*
> **Young woman (twenty-four):** But we are always taught, you know, in the transit school we are taught that religion (*chö*) is important, and that material things cannot bring you real happiness.
> **Young male newcomer:** But don't you see the monks in Dharamsala, flying here and flying there, they say they are spreading the dharma but really they are getting rich and maybe His Holiness doesn't even know what they are doing.
> **Young woman (twenty-four):** This is just gossip.
> **Elderly man:** Money comes and goes, this is the teaching of the dharma, you should not be attached to possessions.

Yet, despite tensions related to income disparities and the lack of opportunities in exile, India-born Tibetan youth feel more at home in India than publicised messages of longing for the homeland suggest. Tibetan students and monks relish Bollywood films and enjoy gorging in the restaurants of Lower Dharamsala. This was pointed out to me on many occasions, including during one *losar* evening, when a group of teenage Tibetan students planning their day's outing to Kotwali bazaar and visits to the toys and hair accessory shops, exclaimed, 'India is the happiest place!'[3]

For many first-generation refugees, India is a place of cherished memories and opportunities. In Gangkyi, one can often find three generations of Tibetans eating dinner in front of a Bollywood film recommended by elders because it reminds them of their 'youth'. Gangkyi's intellectual elites, a great number of which are trained at the Central Institute of Higher Tibetan Studies in Sarnath, have strong views about Indo-Tibetan friendship: to them, India is the home of Buddhism and a patron to Tibetans. As one teacher stated: 'India is our spiritual home. Buddhism came from India; we translated many texts from Indian masters. India gave us refuge, we are safe here. Many of us speak Hindi, and people from the school at Sarnath also know Sanskrit! So you see, we are really at home!'

Tibetans therefore have contrasting views of Dharamsala. To some, like first generation refugees, Dharamsala is a temporary home that has become a permanent one. To others, such as newcomers, it is a town where opportunities are slim. I return to this problem in Chapters 5 and 6, and look at additional differences between 'old-timers' and 'newcomers'.

Managing health in exile: medical pluralism

Tibetan exiles' stories are entangled with tales of medical neglect and discrimination. Tibetan political prisoners suffer extreme abuse in Chinese prisons: beatings, electric shocks, shackling, and multiple forms of torture are commonly reported by Human Rights Watch and Amnesty International.[4] The perilous flight over the Himalayas to the Nepalese border takes on average one month, increasing up to three months for escapees from Kham and Amdo. During this journey, refugees incur injury and frostbite, and many arrive in Nepal gravely malnourished. They also face forced repatriation, robbery, and sexual assault by Nepali border patrols and opportunistic middlemen.

When they reach Dharamsala, refugees are usually accommodated in the reception centre financed by the Dalai Lama's relief fund (see Figure 2.2). This lasts for about fifteen days on average. During this crucial period, a nurse or doctor from the biomedical hospital gives new refugees an initial health check. A government official takes down their details and the story of their escape. Their basic needs are 'assessed', and an audience with the Dalai Lama is scheduled before they are relocated to educational facilities or to other Indian

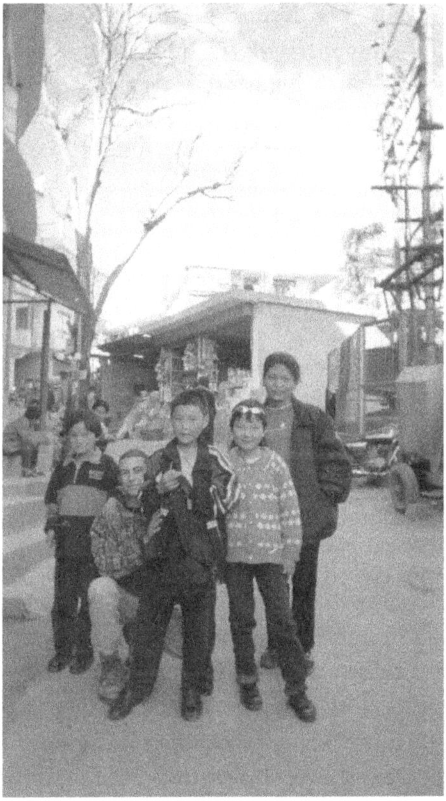

Figure 2.2: Young Tibetan newcomers outside the Tibetan Reception Centre in Dharamsala on the day before their 'relocation' to local exile schools. (Photo: Audrey Prost, 2001)

settlements. The refugees are given a 'starting fund' and second-hand clothes.[5]

Although Tibetans benefit from the protection of the United Nations High Commission for Refugees upon arrival in Nepal, in practice, the abuse of Tibetans crossing the border into exile is widespread and commonly reported by human rights agencies in Kathmandu and Dharamsala. In general, the health of newcomers upon arrival in India is poor. Many Tibetans from the rural regions of Kham and Amdo do not have access to primary care, and are consequently not vaccinated for diseases such as TB, polio, or typhoid until their arrival in Kathmandu or Dharamsala's reception centres. A great number of Tibetan children who reach the exile schools in India do not have a BCG scar.[6] Reports quote numerous testimonies of discrimination in access to health-care facilities, with Tibetans being forced to put down exorbitant deposits to enter a 'public' hospital (Tibet Information Network, 2002). In Lhasa, unemployment, discrimination, and social anomie reportedly exert a toll on Tibetans' health (Adams et al., 2005). Jamyang Norbu vividly expresses this pervasive feeling of helplessness:

> People don't become alcoholics for the love of it. There are certain conditions where everything seems to be hopeless. And the only rosy thing in life is what you see in that bottle. Tibetans are coming to that, and I don't want to say it in many ways, because the official propaganda, even among Tibetans in exile … is that things are improving, we can get along with the Chinese, and something wonderful is going to happen, it's just around the corner. I don't see that at all. I see a broken people; broken by the Cultural Revolution; broken by what's happening now.[7]

Medical pluralism is the norm in Dharamsala (see Table 2.1). The majority of exiles interviewed in this study subscribed to the view that biomedical and traditional Tibetan medical systems are complementary, and few doubted the benefits of using both concurrently. Individuals would often juggle a number of practitioners and treatments over the course of a lengthy illness. Typically, Tibetans explained that they visited the Delek (biomedical) hospital and the Mentsikhang (traditional) clinic for different types of illnesses: they would go to Delek for readily identifiable biomedical disorders, and to

Table 2.1: Medical Pluralism in Dharamsala

Practitioners	Practice	Numbers	Visited by	Links with
Traditional Tibetan doctors	In Mentsikhang clinics or privately	Forty-seven Mentsikhang branch clinics in India and Nepal	All, but mostly elderly patients	Biomedical hospitals
Biomedically trained doctors	Delek Hospital	Four in Delek Hospital	All, with great numbers of TB patients	Mentsikhang
Mopas (diviners)	Privately	As many as thirty practitioners in Dharamsala	All, including older refugees and newcomers	Officially none, but critically influence patients' choice of treatment
Lay diviners and astrologers	Privately, on markets	At least five lay practitioners in Dharamsala		

the Mentsikhang for problems that fit the description of Tibetan humoral disorders, usually chronic illnesses.

Tibetan medicine has never been legalised in India, although Ayurveda and homeopathy have been granted special status within the Indian national medical system.[8] This means that Tibetan medical treatments are provided for a fee in traditional clinics, though sometimes at subsidised rates for refugees on low income. With the growing popularity of Tibetan medicine abroad however, Tibetan practitioners are working towards the standardisation of medical training and production in order to achieve legal status.

Other key agents in the medical landscape of Dharamsala are religious practitioners. Some of these have trained in medicine in addition to their monastic education. There are also lay diviners, often referred to as *mopa*. Learned monks and lay diviners regularly perform rituals such as *mo* (oracular reading of dice or prayer beads) at the request of individuals or families.[9] *Mopa* are called upon in cases of serious illness, both to identify causes and to prescribe an appropriate course of therapeutic action, whether biomedical or traditional.

The *mopa*'s divination sometimes relates the illness to possession of the sufferer by a malevolent spirit (*don*), and prescribes the appropriate exorcism. This may involve a ritual purification of the home, or spiritual practices such as recitations of sacred texts and offerings. According to one teacher at the Mentsikhang, after conducting a *mo* to ascertain whether a *don* has caused the illness, the diviner judges the seriousness of the illness involved. If the illness is a mere weakness, fever, or cold, the patient is given a charm to hang around the neck or to keep within the home. These charms can be amulets consisting of pieces of paper with a protective mantra or symbol of the demon's enemy. If the illness is more severe, however, the diviner makes an effigy of the spirit out of clay or bread paste (*ku lu*, or literally, 'ransom offering'). The spirit, fooled by the effigy, recognises itself and, by entering its own representation, is trapped in it. The effigy is then burnt or buried, and purifying rituals are performed in the sick person's house. There are renowned diviners in Dharamsala, Dehra Dun, and Clement Town, who perform divinations and *lu* rituals. On occasion, Mentsikhang astrology students and teachers are commissioned to make amulets containing the names of particular deities.[10]

According to the same Mentsikhang teacher however, the work of traditional Tibetan physicians is becoming increasingly dissociated with divination, at least in Dharamsala. The enrolment of ritual specialists to carry out purification rituals is not dealt with by Mentsikhang but rather through monasteries (in Gangkyi, for instance, monks from the nearby Gadong monastery perform funerary rites and *don* exorcisms).[11] It is also worth noting that astrology is becoming less popular as a subject of study among young Tibetans, in contrast to medicine. Overall, this suggests a gradual decline in ritual activity related to spirit attacks.

Exiled Tibetans also consult Mentsikhang and independent astrologers (*tsipa*) for advice on suitable dates for weddings and rituals associated with funerals or don expurgations. The Dalai Lama himself is known to perform *mo* divinations, and a number of monks in Dharamsala are solicited on a regular basis to help families in need.

The presence of diviners in the medical landscape of Dharamsala is an enduring and important feature. In practice, it actualises a major link between Buddhist conceptions of illness, medical aetiologies, and therapeutic management: diviners are often the gatekeepers of therapeutic action, directing sufferers to specific practitioners and prescribing appropriate therapeutic strategies. One may speculate that the great number of therapeutic options available in Dharamsala forces individuals into difficult choices, and often leads them to consult 'independent' agents such as religious and lay diviners in order to finalise decisions. In the following chapter, I examine subjective perceptions of health among Tibetan exiles, and specifically the notion of exile as a 'pathogenic' environment.

Notes

1. UNHCR. 2003. India: Information on Tibetan refugees and settlements. http://www.unhcr.org/cgi-bin/texis/vtx/home/opendoc.htm?tbl=RSDCOI&page=research&id=3f51f90821
2. The only other alternative is settlement housing, for which a minor rent is paid, or staff quarters, which are only given to retired civil servants and workers of academic institutes. One CTA civil servant further explained that, 'even if one doesn't own his/her house, one has to pay a small tax which is deducted straight from one's salary': *'so so'i khang pa yod na 'khral nyung nyung sbrad dgos red ani gla cha nas bcad kyi yod red'*. The tax is paid to the Tibetan government in exile as a more or less obligatory contribution (there is no sanction for non-payment but it is expected as a token of loyalty and cooperation with the government), as the CTA is not formally allowed to raise taxes.
3. *'Rgya gar skyid shos red!'*
4. See Amnesty International Report (2005) on China. For an account of the Tibetan Torture Survivor Programme in Dharamsala, see Mercer et al., 2005.
5. This is a contentious issue. I spoke with some newcomers who argued that the government in exile can no longer cope with the influx of new refugees and that new refugees are now being offered 4,000 rupees to make the journey back to Tibet. However, most 'older settlers' deny this, and Gangkyi workers are simply outraged at the suggestion that new refugees are being turned away.
6. The Tibet Information Network's (2002) report, entitled *Delivery and Deficiency: Health and Health Care in Tibet*, states that 'the Tibet Autonomous Region has the highest rate of tuberculosis in the PRC.'
7. In 'Dreams of Tibet' Frontline Documentary Transcripts: http://www.pbs.org/wgbh/pages/frontline/shows/tibet/interviews/norbu1.html.
8. This was enshrined in the 1970 Central Council of Indian Medicine Act.

9. The practice of *mo* is said to have its origins in the pre-Buddhist Bonpo tradition of Tibet (Stein, 1972). As such, *mo* was part of popular religion and practised by lay and Bon diviners before being appropriated by tantric specialists (*nagpa*). In the Indian exile, mo divinations are carried out by individual lay 'specialists' or monks refered to as *mopa*. The most common forms of *mo* are the throwing of dice and manipulation of the *tengwa* (prayer beads), a practice called *teng mo*.
10. One male astrology student reported making amulets containing the name of the deity Hayagrîva to ward off the ill intent of the controversial deity Shugden. Shugden worship has been strongly condemned by the Dalai Lama and the Tibetan government in exile. For an exhaustive account of the rise of the Shugden cult, see Dreyfus (1999).
11. For more on *don* in Dharamsala, see Calkowski (1985).

Chapter 3
The Pathogenic Nature of Exile

When I first arrived in Dharamsala, my aim was to research the health-care 'cultures' of Tibetan exiles. However, following discussions with Tibetan patients at the biomedical hospital and in the Mentsikhang, my initial concern with health-care evolved into a broader preoccupation with physical and mental well-being as experienced by exiles. It soon became apparent that Tibetans' conceptions of health were linked to issues encompassing the environment, politics, and social welfare.

An unhealthy environment

One of the first themes to emerge in interviews conducted in 2001 was a strong preoccupation with the exile environment. Tibetans felt at risk from dangerous microorganisms (*bu*) in food and water, and assailed by air pollution (*lung tsogpa*) caused by the increasing amount of motorised traffic in Dharamsala. Many believed that the exile environment was itself a health hazard to Tibetans, who fell ill because of the exposure to unknown bacteria, parasites, and pollutants.

Pema, a 16-year-old female student from the Tibetan Children's Village said:

> I think [that] what most affects us here is that they are destroying the environment. Building hotels everywhere, making roads that never get finished, really they are polluting ... In Tibet it is not like that. If you look at pictures of Tibet, you know, the rural areas, the sky is always deep blue, the mountains are very, you know, pure ... Here it's like living in Delhi, but on the mountain. But maybe Tibet has changed so much it is also very polluted. I think the Chinese are polluting a lot.*

This was echoed in the words of a Tibet-born 25-year-old male Mentsikhang student: 'We can't find the plants to make our traditional medicines here. In Tibet, we have everything we need. In the big cities like Lhasa or Nagchu, it is quite polluted now, but, if you go on a trip to the countryside, it is so beautiful, very pure.' Phuntsog, a McLeod shop-owner, explained how water supplies essential to his business regularly became 'contaminated':

> I use this water to make curd [*sho*] for sale. But it always gets dirty and then people get sick. Even I get sick drinking it. Maybe it is contaminated earth in the water or maybe some organisms [*bu*]. We called a lama to come and say prayers, and the contamination [*drip*] went away. Now it's back. I can't sell my curd, this place is too dirty, I will have to move.

Many Tibetans viewed the exile environment as pathogenic. Pollutants and dangerous 'microorganisms' brought endless stomach problems and diarrhoea. On the other hand, when I asked India-born Tibetans about prevalent illnesses in Tibet, many told me their homeland was free of the diseases endemic to the subcontinent because of its high altitude and dry, cold climate. This belief is reflected in the following words from a retired Tibet-born soldier: 'In Tibet the wind is always blowing and it is the highest place in the world, therefore there really is no disease.'[1] A Tibetan woman in her forties who travelled regularly between India and Tibet told me:

> You know, what they say is really true, the water in Tibet is like the milk in India, it is so rich and wonderful, and the meat tastes like ... you have never tasted anything like it ... Whenever I go back there, at once I feel better, you will not believe me, but I feel like I am ten years younger.

Many Tibetans in the local biomedical hospital and the Mentsikhang had experienced new 'Indian' disorders such as malaria or dysentery upon their arrival in India. According to them, most refugees got sick after arriving in India. Furthermore, many exiles reported suffering from long-term chronic conditions, which they believed were caused by their exposure to the Indian environment. One Tibetan student explained her view of the relationship between exile and illness succinctly: 'If this place doesn't agree with you, wounds and diseases will come.'[2] Through this comment, she expressed a belief in the direct relationship between the exile environment and adverse health outcomes.

The explanations given by Tibetans for prevalent diseases in the community included concerns about changes in the environment, diet, and social circumstances. Table 3.1 summarises the findings of short structured interviews in which patients from the Mentsikhang and Delek Hospital were asked which diseases were prevalent in exile. I interviewed thirty-eight individuals visiting Delek and thirty-six at the Mentsikhang. Thirty-five were women and thirty-nine were men. All were above sixteen years old. The majority of patients were aged between thirty and sixty (fifty-four respondents out of seventy-four), and a sizeable proportion had been born in Tibet (fifty-seven per cent).

Following the initial small survey presented in Table 3.1, I sought to understand local explanations for prevalent disorders (see Table 3.2).

This small survey showed that explanations for prevalent disorders centred mainly on environmental determinants of health: changes in

Table 3.1: Disorders considered 'prevalent' in the exile community; (B) indicates that the person interviewed felt the disorder had a biomedical aetiology; (T) a traditional Tibetan one; (B & T) suggests that both may be valid.

Tibetan term	English term	MTK	At Delek
Dokhog shelwa (B)	Diarrhoea	2	22
Chinni natsa (B & T)	Diabetes	6	17
Tibi natsa (B)	Tuberculosis	36	38
Champa (B & T)	Cold/influenza	23	10
Tumbu'i natsa (B & T)	Arthritis, rheumatism	25	16
Chin ne (B & T)	Liver disorders	28	15
Dzene (B & T)	Leprosy	12	10
AIDS (B)	AIDS	12	19
Tragshe (B)	High blood pressure	32	31
Go ne (B & T)	Headaches	4	19
Cancer (B)	Cancer	30	36
Powa'i natsa (B & T)	Stomach disease	32	29
Kel ne (T)	Kidney disease	30	12
Nyingi natsa (B & T)	Heart disease	15	35

Table 3.2: Explanations for prevalent disorders (thirty-six patients from Mentsikhang and thirty-eight patients from Delek Hospital).

Disorder Category	Causes (English)	Causes (Tibetan)	% (No.) MTK	% (No.) Delek Hospital
Dokhog shelwa (diarrhoea)	Unclean water	*chu tsog pa*	61 (22)	68 (26)
	Insect/bacteria	*'bu*	47 (17)	89 (34)
	Rotten/bad foods	*Kala rulwa*	44 (16)	29 (11)
Chinni natsa	Fatty/oily foods	*kala numpa*	89 (32)	66 (25)
	Overeating	*kala tel sawa*	86 (31)	79 (30)
	Tripa 'disorder'	*tripa*	80 (29)	58 (22)
	Heredity (descent)	*dung gyu*	36 (13)	66 (25)
	Karma (past actions)	*le*	14 (5)	18 (7)
Tibi natsa (TB)	Infectious bu	*gowa'i bu*	92 (33)	100 (38)
	Living with TB patients	*tibi nepa nyamdu de*	72 (26)	63 (24)
	Irregular/insufficient eating	*cu med se che*	72 (26)	29 (11)
	Karma (past actions)	*le*	28 (10)	16 (6)
Champa (cold)	Being in cold and damp places	*sache dangmo dang she tsen do*	97 (35)	84 (32)
	Cold climate	*namshi tangmo*	94 (34)	97 (37)
	Contagion from family or neighbours	*nangmi/kimtse go ne gyabpa*	22 (8)	58 (22)
Drumbu'i natsa (arthritis, rheumatism)	Being in cold and damp places	*nangmi/kimtse go ne gyabpa*	86 (31)	71 (27)
	Cold foods	*kala tangmo*	83 (30)	60 (23)
	Heat and cold disorder	*tangwa dang tsawa la sogpa'i dugnyel*	44 (16)	24 (9)
	Karma (past actions)	*le*	50 (18)	31 (12)
Dzene (leprosy)	Living in poor, bad conditions	*ulpo, dugcha de*	75 (27)	89 (34)
	Karma	*le*	36 (13)	37 (14)
	Lepers	*dze nepa*	28 (10)	47 (18)
	The condition of having *chu ser nag po/tripa*	*chu ser nag po dang mkhris pa*	17 (6)	8 (3)
Cancer	Heredity	*dung gyu*	5 (2)	24 (9)
	Change in food habits	*shelug rolgyur*	19 (7)	29 (11)
	Changing from habitual place and climate	*sacha dang namshi gyur*	47 (17)	55 (21)
	Old age	*geka*	80 (29)	60 (23)
	Karma	*le*	13 (5)	8 (3)
AIDS	Sexual intercourse	*drugi don tonpa*	58 (21)	53 (20)
	Karma	*le*	44 (16)	10 (4)
	Virus	*dug ca na skye dan phra rab*	33 (12)	42 (16)
Tragshe (high blood pressure)	Salty and rich foods	*kala numpa*	89 (32)	100 (38)
	Heredity	*dung gyu*	42 (15)	42 (16)
	Alcohol	*chang, arak*	61 (22)	66 (38)

Table 3.2 (continued)

Disorder Category	Causes (English)	Causes (Tibetan)	% (No.) MTK	% (No.) Delek Hospital
Go ne (headaches)	*Tripa* imbalance	*tripa*	75 (27)	30 (16)
	Hot climate, being under the sun	*namshi tsapo, nyi ma 'og sdod*	83 (30)	68 (26)
	Use of alcohol or strong tea	*chang, arak, cha karpo tungwa*	69 (25)	58 (22)
	Heart–*lung* imbalance	*nying lung*	33 (12)	48 (17)
	Demon/spirit influence	*don*	11 (4)	21 (8)
Phowa'i natsa (stomach problem)	Cold foods	*kala tangmo*	58 (21)	26 (10)
	Unclean foods	*kala ma tsang*	79 (30)	84 (32)
	Unclean water	*chu tsogpa*	97 (35)	87 (33)
	Hot or spicy food	*kala tsapo–kyurpo sawa*	36 (13)	21 (8)
kel ne (kidney problem)	Cold climate	*namshi tangmo*	80 (29)	66 (25)
	beygen/lung disorder	*beygen, lung*	55 (20)	44 (17)
	lung/tripa disorder	*lung, tripa*	39 (14)	5 (2)
	Sweet foods	*kala ngarmo*	36 (13)	16 (6)
	Alcohol	*chang, arak*	28 (10)	5 (2)
	Cold foods	*kala tangmo*	39 (14)	24 (9)
Nyingi natsa (heart problem)	*rlung*	*lung*	33 (12)	34 (13)
	Fatty foods	*kalag numpa*	83 (30)	68 (26)
	High blood pressure	*tragshe*	86 (31)	79 (30)
Chin ne (liver problem)	Fatty foods	*kala numpa*	69 (25)	42 (16)
	'Brown bad kan'	*beygen mugpo*	55 (21)	53 (20)
	Hot spicy foods	*kala tsapo*	72 (26)	53 (20)
	mkhrispa disorder	*tripa*	53 (19)	17 (45)
	Alcohol	*chang, arak*	83 (30)	84 (32)
	Hepatitis	*hepatitis*	36 (13)	63 (24)
Lungi natsa (wind disorder)	Worry, anxiety	*semtel chepa*	69 (25)	79 (30)
	Financial problems	*ngulgi nyogta-semtel*	86 (31)	84 (32)
	Sadness	*kyo ngelwa*	64 (23)	47 (18)
	Family problems	*shetsang tsopa – nyogta*	39 (14)	50 (19)
	Changing from 'hot' to 'cold' place	*sacha tsawa ne silwar gyur*	42 (15)	50 (19)
	Unbalanced activity levels, unhappy life	*tsetsul ma nyom, tse tsul ma kyi*	50 (18)	58 (22)
	Demon, spirit influence	*don*	17 (6)	8 (3)
Tripa'i natsa (bile disorder)	Hot climate	*namshi tangmo*	15 (42)	10 (4)
	Hot foods	*kalag tsapo*	50 (18)	34 (13)
	Fatty foods	*kalag numpa*	61 (22)	53 (20)
Lo'i natsa (lung problems)	Dirty air (pollution, (esp. car pollution)	*lung tsogpa*	83 (30)	89 (34)
	lung	*lung*	19 (7)	10 (4)
	Smoking	*tama tenpa*	77 (28)	81 (31)
	Taking snuff powder	*nata tung*	14 (5)	29 (11)
	Incense burning	*sang sur*	17 (6)	3 (1)

the environment, air quality, and living 'in poor conditions' were perceived as the most common causes of disease in the settlement. Patients reported varied aetiologies for prevalent disorders: explanations often incorporated both biomedical references (e.g., 'viruses') and traditional Tibetan concepts (e.g., *lung*). There were also numerous allusions to psychosocial factors (sadness, worry, anxiety) and to karma. Evidently, the environment of exile itself was thought to be responsible for many ailments in the community.

Exile as pathogenic

Findings from this survey and subsequent interviews suggest that many Tibetans view the exile environment as pathogenic. For example, India's hot climate, the way foods seemed to rot, the lack of wind, and the lack of space were thought to contribute to the rise of *tripa* and *lung* disorders. As a form of socially sanctioned traditional knowledge, traditional Tibetan medicine is employed to counteract the disruption caused by environmental, behavioural, and dietary changes among exiles. Tibetan medicine privileges multifactorial understandings of disease and links disorders to both the environment and the psychological state of individuals.

Tibetan medicine also provides therapies to deal with the disorders of exile. In recent years, there has been a booming demand for prophylactic traditional medicines such as the blessed pills (*mani rilbu*) blessed by lamas and distributed during religious ceremonies in Dharamsala's main temple. These pills are part of the broader category of empowered sacred substances called *jinden*, which also include seeds or waters blessed by high lamas on ritual occasions. *Jinden* substances such as *mani rilbu* are kept in homes for months and distributed to friends and family. They are consumed by family members whenever illness occurs, first preventively, and then sometimes as a complement to biomedical medications. When three members of a family I knew fell ill after feasting during *losar*, for example, the female household head promptly produced a cocktail of aspirin and Tibetan pills which were taken together, literally 'crushed one straight after another' in the same glass of boiled water. The *jinden* can also be taken when a special blessing is required. For instance, students take the pills before government examinations to help them cope with tiredness and endow them with the blessings of lamas. Traditional empowered substances like *jinden* are used as prophylactic medicines, helping Tibetans protect themselves against the vicissitudes of a hostile exile environment.

In addition to the arsenal of *jinden*, exiles also attribute prophylactic and curative properties to substances that come from Tibet, perhaps because such substances have acquired a strong affective meaning in the diaspora (see Table 3.3). For example, the traditional belief in the medicinal properties of butter and milk is often discussed in the context of exile: 'In Tibet, water tastes like milk,' I was once told by an elderly nun, or another variation: 'The milk in India tastes like the water from Tibet.' Foods and drinks from Tibet are seen as especially nutritious and vitality-enhancing: yak meat, scarce in exile, is said to have a richer and more pungent taste than any meat available in India. There is a homology between the use of food brought from Tibet and that of *jinden*: both are considered to have curative, protective, and revitalising qualities. Thus offering food from Tibet may be considered a virtuous act much in the same way as the gift of *jinden* is. Other protective objects include Tibetan religious or medical books, which are often kept in the home for protection and a wide variety of substances (see Figure 3.1) that are infused the bio-moral qualities of Tibet, like dried yak meat, or of persons, like *jinden*.

Table 3.3: Medicinal and Protective Substances

Medicinal products	Medicinal substances	Protective objects and substances	Vitality enhancing foods
Pills (*rilbu*)	Herbs (*ngo*)	Talismans (*sungwa*)	Foods imported from Tibet or Bhutan, e.g., cheese or yak meat (*churwa*, *yak*)
Powders, preparations and pastes	Minerals (*sater*)	Blessed pills (*mani rilbu*)	Vitality enhancing substances: butter (*mar*), milk (*oma*), and water (*chu*) from Tibet
		jinden	Foods given to attendees at the temple, e.g., biscuits, fruits (*tsog*)

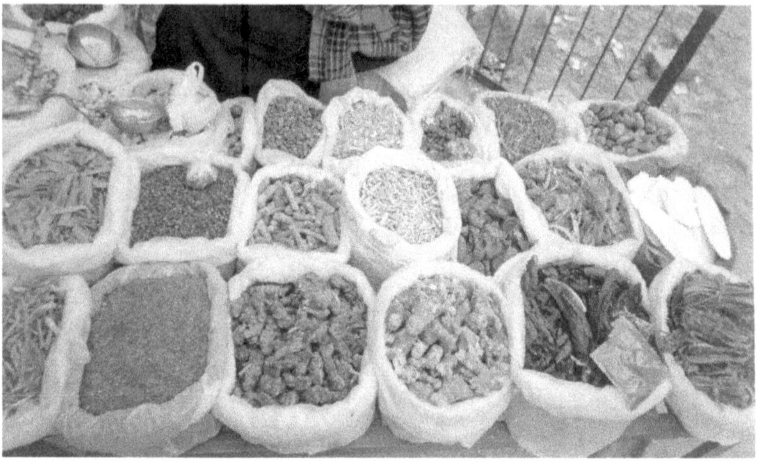

Figure 3.1: Tibetan woman selling medicinal substances in Dharamsala: tree barks, ginger roots, garlic and cuttlefish shells. (Photo: Audrey Prost, 2000)

Armed with substances such as *mani rilbu* and *jinden*, exiles confront an exile environment which they often view as pathogenic. Tibetan medicine thus plays a crucial role in maintaining collective health in exile, not only through the private consultations given by Mentsikhang practitioners, but also through the collective distribution of blessed or empowered substances. In the next section, I examine the social impact of exile as described by Tibetan refugees, as well as the connections made between social change and health at a local level.

The social impact of exile

The radical social and economic changes experienced by Tibetans with the move to India in the 1960s have had a very real impact on health and morale in the community. As Seidman (1997) describes it: 'A feeling of despair grips Tibetan youth who have difficulty finding employment within their own communities ... [They] either move to large urban cities which may only have a small Tibetan community or none at all; or they attempt to emigrate, which is almost impossible; or they stay in their own communities and are under-utilised.' Many Tibetans think that, in addition to environmental factors, the main causes of ill-health in the community are poverty and social isolation. The lack of opportunity, idleness, and despair associated with exile are seen as conducive to disease.

A 36-year-old housewife from McLeod Ganj spoke about the problems faced by young people in the community:

> When we came to Dharamsala we had nothing. Just a stove, you know, some blankets, and that's it. Nothing … But we worked very hard, and we tried to stay healthy, tried to follow His Holiness' advice with our body, speech, and mind. But now I am scared for these young boys and girls. So many girls, trying to look good, follow fashion, even to look Indian! They become ill because they try to look like models … And also young boys, newcomers ... Many go into monasteries and they just become ill because there is so much TB there. Young people have a difficult life. For us it is easier now, though we are sad because we cannot go back to Tibet. We have His Holiness, we work, we have friends. What do they have? No jobs, everyone is trying to go to Ari-lo [America].*

A Tibetan musician born in India spoke about the ambivalent feelings of young people towards their Tibetan identity:

> I can't bear to stay here sometimes. Nothing changes. Every year, the same thing … *Losar*, *Monlam*, we celebrate the birthdays of Karmapa and Gyalwa Rinpoche. It's the same [thing], the same … Of course it is good for us to do all this, but from my point of view sometimes it's … it's like a show. Everybody is saying how great Tibetans are, but if you go on the circumambulation path in the morning, then you hear what people are saying about each other, 'Oh look, he has more money now,' 'Oh, she bought a house there.' We have nothing to do, so we gossip about each other. And we try to stay busy. Some of my friends it drives them crazy and they want to go away, go to Tibet, go to America, Canada, anywhere. *

The uncertainty of exile takes its toll on young people's morale, and many newcomers dream of returning to Tibet or travelling further abroad. Dorjee, a young newcomer, explained:

> I have friends who go back to Tibet. Almost every week, we bring one of them to the bus stop to say goodbye. Often we cry because we know we will never see each other again. But the most important thing is that, every night we stay up and we talk about going back to Tibet, about what we should do. Every night … It is a happy thing because

> we are friends, but we also know that we cannot stay here. There are no jobs for us ... Some of us have lost everything: family, girlfriends, work.

A young newcomer who worked as an assistant in the pharmacy department of the Mentsikhang also talked about feeling like an outsider in the exile community because of his upbringing in Chinese-occupied Tibet:

> I don't know ... I didn't think it [exile] would be so difficult. I was told I had family here, but when I came to India I found out they have moved to Bylakuppe [South India]. So I don't really have relatives here, I have never met them. I was lucky to find this job, that is true. But back in Tibet I was earning more and I had family, friends. People my age who were born in India all have their own friends, so I mostly stay with people from Lhasa. Sometimes we go and have noodle soup in the restaurant and there is a Chinese programme that we like to watch, but people, how do you say, they look at us. We speak Chinese, we understand it, and they don't like that.

More politically minded Tibetans viewed ill health as directly related to community welfare, and, more specifically, to religious observance, as a 'welfare officer'[3] (WO) explained in 2002:

> **AP:** What do you think is the most important thing for Tibetan people's health, here, in Dharamsala?
> **WO:** His Holiness [the Dalai Lama] prays for our health, the health of the Tibetan people. This is one of the most important things. Of course we have a good hospital, we have Mentsikhang, but the most important thing is that we are religious. His Holiness gives us guidance on how to lead a good life, a healthy life. If everyone followed his advice we would all be well.
> **AP:** What about young people?
> **WO:** Especially young people! They should follow His Holiness. Old people are very religious, that is normal, but normal people too, instead of always thinking about their problems, they should think of others, just like His Holiness says.*

Other young people identified militant activism as a way to show their patriotism and attachment to the Tibetan cause, but also as an activity that gave meaning to their lives. One regular Tibetan hunger striker living between Delhi and Dharamsala said that political activism kept him 'sane':

> If I don't do anything about this situation, then I feel powerless, I feel unhappy. Doing hunger strikes is something very powerful, very pure, something that great people like Mahatma Gandhi used to fight injustice. When I do a strike I feel good in my mind. Of course, I feel hungry [laughs], but I feel good in my mind. We have lots of supporters, people who believe in us you know, they count on us. When you are doing it, you know you have a goal, and this is what you live for. Even if His Holiness does not like hunger strikes, we always get in the newspapers, we are shouting 'Free Tibet' high and loud. This makes me feel good. Not like the politicians in Dharamsala doing nothing and taking dollars. I think it's better to do hunger strikes than to do drugs. I am doing this for Tibet, for my friends, for my parents.*

Different perspectives on health and well-being emerge from these accounts. For some, well-being is fostered by proximity to the Dalai Lama and religious practice. For others, it is maintained through political activism. Others yet, including older Tibetans, feel that the lack of opportunities in exile has generated idleness and cynicism, which then leads to unhealthy behaviour such as drug use. These accounts illustrate some of the different factors that influence people's understandings of health: proximity to family and a network of friends, religious observance, and political activism are seen as sources of meaning and therefore as catalysts for 'healthy behaviour'. On the other hand, as I explore further in the next chapter, newcomers often report feeling alienated by older settlers. The fact that many have grown in Chinese-occupied Tibet makes them ideal targets for accusations of spying and bringing illnesses into the settlement.

Notes

1. *'Bod la lung rbad de gtsang ma dang sa 'dzam gling nas mtho shos yin tsang na tsa 'dra min 'dra yod ma red.'* Although many exiled Tibetans claim that tuberculosis did not exist in Tibet before the Chinese invasion, there are strong reasons to doubt this. First, Tibet has long entertained trade relations with China, India, Nepal, and other Central Asian countries, making its isolation from diseases like TB highly doubtful. Secondly, TB is now reported as endemic in the Tibetan Autonomous Region.
2. *'Sa cha 'di ma 'phrod na, sma dang na tsha 'dra min 'dra yong gi red.'*
3. Welfare officers are elected civil servants who play an important role in providing key services to the community, such as arranging gas provision or helping families with sick relatives with transport to health-care facilities.

Chapter 4
From 'Old-timers' to 'Newcomers': Social Inequalities in the Diaspora

> One day a newcomer arrived in Dharamsala, and visited the library. Seeing the great work done by people there and how many foreigners it is attracting, he decides that he too can make some profit and opens up a tourist bureau in McLeod. From there he takes tourists to Bodh Gaya and the Bodhi tree, where he says: 'Here the Buddha spent many years, pillar cutting [*ka ba bcad*].'
> [In a religious context, *ka ba bcad* means 'eliminating suffering'. The newcomer has given it a literal meaning: 'pillar cutting'], which is interpreted as a characteristic sign of religious ignorance. (Government worker's joke, January 2001)

This chapter deals with socio-economic inequalities between first- and second-generation refugees (old-timers), and recently arrived Tibetans (newcomers). First, I explore the support networks available to 'old-timers' and how these impact on health-seeking behaviour. Secondly, I turn to the newcomers' predicament and investigate their views on support and health in exile.

The importance of social ties: old-timers

The Tibetan community in India is composed of a heterogeneous range of social groups, encompassing first-generation refugees, second- or third-generation India-born Tibetans, and newcomers (Bhatia et al., 2002a). First-generation Tibet-born refugees now represent only approximately 35 per cent of the exile population. The economic constraints of exile may have 'physically' reduced Tibetan homesteads to nuclear households, but, in practice, these 'downsized' families are in contact with relatives in Dharamsala and other settlements. Although they may not be co-residents with members of their extended family, couples often live in close proximity to their relatives within the settlements. Moreover, strong informal networks involving friends acting as helpers (*rogpa*) supplement family support networks.

Social ties that involve the reciprocation of services on an informal basis are particularly important and are often referred to as providing *rogpa*, which literally means 'companionship'. *Rogpa* is the company and assistance that family and friends give each other on a daily basis. Being a *rogpa* can involve accompanying a relative or a friend on a shopping errand, or helping a sick person in everyday activities. More than help, *rogpa* qualifies a way of 'being with' or 'shadowing' another person, sometimes in very practical ways: carrying things, or 'simply being there' and guarding the safety of a companion through one's presence.[1] Three women from Dharamsala summarised the uses of *rogpa*:

> **Young female newcomer**: I never talk to monks on my own, I am too scared. They are very important and they know a lot of people. Foreigners talk to them like they are old friends, but we know who they are, we use honorific language.
> **Young female newcomer (2):** When I go to the market, I always take a friend, a *rogpa*. We can sit in the car together and talk, nobody will bother us. If I go on my own, people talk, sometimes Indian men you know they sit very close to you in the car and they put their hand on your leg and you have to shout. When you have *rogpa* it is easier.
> **Older female resident:** What is there to say, it is just a woman's thing.

For my girlfriends and their mothers, the inclusive group of *rogpa* encompassed friends and family whom it was socially safe to mingle with. One should adopt a certain amount of caution in dealing with strangers or persons of markedly higher status, and exercise prudence to avoid behaving innapropriately. One India-born Tibetan exile woman quoted a proverb to explain that it was not always easy to know people's true intentions: 'The tiger wears his stripes outside, man wears his on the inside.'[2] You cannot tell what a person is really like from their appearance. As one female friend explained after a particularly robust gossip session: 'Reputation is very important in this society.'[3] Providing and having *rogpa* engage one's sense of social awareness.

The geographical proximity of close kin, whether living in the same household or not, is a crucial factor in understanding the dynamics of health-seeking behaviour in Dharamsala. Kin and friendship networks play a critical role in an individual's decisions about whether to start, continue, or abandon a therapeutic course of action. The experiences of family and friends with prevalent illnesses such as tuberculosis or diabetes bear heavily on the way in which relatives manage the course of their own illnesses.

> **Male resident (aged thirty-two):** Well, the first person you talk to about a problem is your wife or your husband, isn't it, before you go and see a doctor ... My wife knows about Tibetan medicine, but she also knows about Western medicine. And she talks [laughs], you know, to many people who are sick, so she knows what everybody does and she gives good advice.
> **Male resident (aged fifty-four):** I talk to my friends. I know some important monks who have diabetes, like me, and they tell me what to do. The doctor only sees you very quickly, doesn't have time to talk.
> **Female resident (aged sixty-one):** If I didn't have my niece and her husband here, I would only go down to Delek Hospital once every three months! Because they are there, I can take a car, they help me and wait for me to come out. This is very important when you have TB because you are weak; sometimes you need people to cook for you or to get your food from the market.
> **Male newcomer (aged twenty-five):** I don't have relatives here, but I have my friends. Last year I became very sad, could not sleep, and got very skinny. My friends each gave some money to buy me Horlicks so I would get better. They also told the Mentsikhang doctor about me so I got some precious pills from there.
> **Female newcomer (aged thirty-one):** My best friend had TB some months ago, and I came to see her at Delek at this time. It is very hard here if you do not have family.

In addition to resources pooled from close neighbourhood ties and kin proximity, many Tibetan refugees I spoke with in Dharamsala have enlarged the traditional circle of close family members to include other distant relatives in India. The term *kimtsang*, which directly designates co-residents, still refers to the extended family. The term *nangmi*, literally the people from 'inside', on the other hand, is traditionally used to designate a 'nuclear family'. However the preferred contemporary term for family relatives is *punkya*, of which the root syllable *pun* may be found in all kinship terms designating relatives of one's own generation, including the members of collateral lines. Same-age geographically distant cross-cousins refer to each other as *punkya* or *punche*, thereby emphasising the closeness of the relationship and the maintenance of kinship bonds despite geographical dislocation. The relationship between exiled paternal and maternal aunts and uncles with their nephews and nieces is also that of *punkya*; it is a close relatioship and ideally involves economic and social support. Paternal uncles and aunts (*a khu* and *a ni*) host their nephews and nieces from other settlements frequently, and often present them with gifts and pocket money. Similarly, family members living abroad will also be referred to as *punkya*. Many families therefore retain close ties to their immediate relatives and attempt to reconstitute geographical proximity and support-giving arrangements, often including more distant relatives in their intimate circle.

Male resident (aged fifty-four): Not just in business, but for everything, I call on family. I have a brother in Delhi, one cousin in Canada, some cousins in South India also. And my sister lives in Nepal. If I travel I go and stay with them, and they come and stay with me as well.
Male resident (aged sixty-seven): I have relatives in Darjeeling, they stayed there after His Holiness left. They often come for the New Year, and when their children go to Delhi they also come and see us. Before, when we were in Tibet we did not see each other often, but now [in India] we need each other!
Female resident (aged sixty-one): In Tibet there were houses with, you know, three generations, and this was good. Now young people do not want to live with old grandparents. It is not only widows in the old people's home, you know; some of them have a family but they do not want to help them. Young people prefer to live alone in houses with their children.
Female newcomer (aged thirty-one): That is not true! We take care of our old grandparents! It is just that here there is not enough space and enough money to do it!
Female resident (aged sixty-one): This is also true ... But *punkya* are the most important thing.

As exile brings the need for strong kin networks, distant relatives who have come to India are brought into the tighter nucleus of close kin, and resources are pooled together. In exile, the terms *punkya* (general term for relatives) and *nangmi* (the 'inner' family circle, literally 'insiders') are conflated: *nangmi* now comes to encompass kin living on the same settlement but outside the extended family's household. Thus two first-generation McLeod families involved in business referred to their relatives living in separate households in McLeod Ganj and in Lower Dharamsala respectively as *nangmi*. On the other hand, the patrilineal cousins of the first family, who lived in Delhi, were referred to as *punkya*. It can therefore be argued that the move to exile has made Tibetans reframe traditional kinship categories to 'draw in' distant relatives into the circle of 'insiders' (*nangmi*) and close family.

Perceptions of health-care

In order to find out more about health-care choices in Dharamsala, I conducted semi-structured interviews with five health-care providers (two doctors and three nurses) from the Delek Hospital and five physicians from the Mentsikhang, as well as with fifteen members of the community.[4] Initial fieldwork in the Delek Hospital showed that a wide variety of groups used biomedical services. Mentsikhang, on the other hand, seemed to be frequented by older Tibetans, many of whom were regular visitors. The interviews confirmed these initial impressions but also brought further nuance to the picture. While newcomers attended the hospital, those who did not live in the city centre found it difficult to travel for outpatient clinics. Many also visited the traditional Tibetan medicine 'camps' set up by Mentsikhang in schools for newcomers.

> **AP:** Have you been to Delek [biomedical hospital]?
> **NF2:** In the hot summer months, many girls get ill with diarrhoea and they have to stay indoors and miss class. The doctors from Delek only come every two weeks so if it's Mentsikhang doctors that come here first then we go to them.
> **N5:** My friend had this problem, appendicitis I think it was … It was the Mentsikhang doctor who found it! They put him in the school car and took him straight to the district hospital because at Delek they cannot cure this.
> **N2:** I like Mentsikhang doctors better, they speak to you in Tibetan, and they check your pulse, and they ask you about food and your mind. That is good …

NF1: It's easy to go to Delek if you live in Dharamsala, but from here it takes too long and nobody wants to take you! So you see whoever comes first.

The older group expressed a strong feeling of attachment to Mentsikhang. Many felt that Tibetan medicine was often more appropriate than biomedicine because it was less invasive:

G: Tibetan medicine is like a dull knife …
GF2: Yes, we say that Tibetan medicine is like a dull knife, and foreign medicine is like a sharp knife, it will get rid of your disease but also cut your finger off!
G: The Mentsikhang is a very good place, doctors are very experienced. Some, look, like His Holiness' s physician, they have come all the way from Tibet. They have seen thousands of patients. They know …
GF1: At Mentsikhang, medicine is very cheap, you do not have to wait for hours, and people talk to you. I go there for [my] arthritis and my husband takes Tibetan medicine for his diabetes. We only go once a month to take the medicine, carry it home, that's it ... We are used to it. Every day, with some boiled water, we take the medicines. It is good for us.
GF2: My son works in the pharmacy at Mentsikhang, so I can go there and get medicines for everyone [laughs]. I also get some *rinchen rilbu* [precious pills] to keep in the house, so, when people are sick, they know they can come to our house, we have *rilbu*!
AP: Would you give Tibetan medicine to a child?
GF2: Of course! Hm … sometimes the pills are very big, so you have to crush them well, but children can take medicine.
G: They say Tibetan medicine can even cure cancer. I don't know, but I hear people say that.
GF2: Tibetan medicine can cure anything because it comes with religion [*chö*]! Religious practice is the strongest thing!

When I asked them about their experiences at Delek Hospital, the older group had varied responses:

G: I never want to go there. Sometimes you have to … Once I had an X-ray of my chest there. I had to wait for a long time.
GF1: I went [there] at the time when my daughter gave birth. She should have given birth at home.
G: It's not clean …
GF2: It is clean, and the nurses are very hard-working. There are many foreign doctors. They don't speak Tibetan, but they work hard. I went once for diarrhoea that didn't stop.

The young handicraft workers and shopowners seldom used health-care facilities, but seemed to prefer Delek. The Mentsikhang was characterised as an institution that provided services for 'old people':

H1: I go to Delek, always. Mentsikhang is for old people. And I only go if I really have to, because it makes you sad to see all these sick people.
AP: Why do you say Mentsikhang is for old people?
H1: [At the Mentsikhang] They are very good for things like stomach problems, lung problems, and old people's problems like bone problems and so on …
HF1: Yes, most old people go to Mentsikhang. We don't have time.
AP: It takes time?
B2: Too much time, you have to talk about your body, and then they take your pulse, you have to take lots of medicine …
HF1: No, not really much time, just time to take the medicine, to prepare it, you know.
HF2: Ah, that's an old people's thing. Crush, crush, crush [*shib, shib, shib*] [laughs]. When I am old I will also go to Mentsikhang.
H2: He he, grandmother!
HF1: The biggest problem for women is breast cancer. Doctors at Mentsikhang do not know about this. I read about it in an Indian magazine. They show you how to look for it so you can do it yourself. Maybe they should learn these things at Mentsikhang!
B1: I go to Mentsikhang because I have a '*tripa*' [bile] problem. But I get tired taking these medicines everyday, maybe I will stop soon. They are very good for long-term, you know 'chronic' conditions, but if you have pain Delek is best.

Many newcomers used both biomedicine and traditional medicine indiscriminately. However, some of them particularly enjoyed talking to traditional practitioners. Many Mentsikhang doctors were born in Tibet and established a good rapport with newcomers. Older people visited Mentsikhang for chronic conditions, and gave traditional Tibetan medicine to their families: some kept Tibetan pills in their house to give to relatives, and advised others on healthy behaviour. Handicraft workers, on the other hand, had little time for traditional Tibetan medicine and viewed going to the hospital as a 'last resort'. Time, financial costs, and the type of condition for which help was sought seemed to be the determinant factors in decision-making.

Not so supported: newcomers

In this section, I return to the health predicaments of 'newcomers', Tibetans who arrived in India from the 1980s onward. The majority of newcomers who arrived in India during that period were born in Kham and Amdo, parts of which have been incorporated into Chinese counties. Having received very little Tibetan education, many speak only Chinese and a Tibetan regional dialect. They come to India unprepared for a confrontation with their more established compatriots: earlier Ü–Tsang refugees often perceive Kham and Amdo newcomers as rustic rural folk. This is made evident from the common references to newcomers as upholding the anachronistic custom of polyandry, being uncultured and violent, or simply *kacha* (Hindi: raw), roguish and unkempt (see Diehl, 1997).

The majority of newcomers are young: 44 per cent of all new refugees coming from Tibet from 1996 to 2001 were between fourteen and twenty-five years old, and 17 per cent were thirteen years old or younger. Many of them were either in monastic training in Tibet, or wished to join monastic institutions in India: 40 per cent of all Tibetan refugees arriving in India between 1996 and 2001 were monks and nuns fleeing religious persecution. This very young population of new Tibetan refugees is motivated by better educational and employment prospects (Klieger, 2002). The reality of exile is often disappointing, however: jobs are scarce and the monasteries over-crowded. As a result, many newcomers go back to Tibet after they have finished their studies, or attempt to migrate further afield in search of better opportunities.

In Dharamsala, a rift is apparent between 'old-timers' and newcomers. Some of the more educated newcomers, such as those originating from Lhasa and its surroundings, accuse old Dharamsala refugees of not knowing how to write or speak Tibetan properly. Some imply that earlier Tibetan refugees and their families have 'bastardised' Tibetan. This, however, represents only a small fraction of the population, and the majority of newcomers are now young and men and women with little education, and who have come to India seeking schooling and employment. In the 1970s, Saklani reported that refugees from Amdo perceived the move to exile as a radical social change, whereas refugees from Ü–Tsang had experienced the shift as less extreme (Saklani, 1984: 109). This further points to the difficulty of Khamdo newcomers in 'finding their feet' in a sometimes unwelcoming exile environment.

Questions of identity and belonging are at the heart of the newcomer/older settler tension. First, earlier refugees tend to see newcomers as immigrants, and thus competition for jobs and sponsorship opportunities. Secondly, newcomers bring with them an image of home that does not always fit with general expectations; for many, they appear rough and unsophisticated, incongruous in Dharamsala's cosmopolitan environment. The following section investigates the dynamics of *rogram* in more detail.

Rogram

Rogram, or 'sponsorship', refers to the money given by outsiders, generally foreigners, to support Tibetans. In exile, providing *rogram* ranges from giving money to using contacts to obtain official papers, invitations to foreign countries, favours, or contacts. Only help from 'sponsors' is considered *rogram*; help received from family members, abroad or in India, does not fall into this category. Many families in Dharamsala receive some form of *rogram* for their children to help them through primary and secondary education, after which studies have to be financed either by the family, or again by foreign sponsors (Prost, 2006b). Newcomers receive an initial 'reception' sum from the Tibetan government in exile to set up home (5,000 rupees), and, if need be, are directed to educational facilities where they can also have board and accommodation. Most newcomers I have spoken with argued that the term *rogram* is specific to exile and to the relationship that foreigners foster with Tibetan refugees. The term 'sponsor' is also used in communication with foreigners, although *rogram* is preferred among Tibetans. In a discussion of the role of aid in the lives of Tibetan refugees, De Voe asserts (1981b: 80, 93):

> The study of the relationships between the givers and receivers or benefactors and beneficiaries attends to the elements of compassion, gratitude and mutual trust theoretically and ideally implicit in this interaction ... Through this relationship, refugees are kept in a

> position of helplessness, and gradually learn to conform to expectations of a 'clientele' of aid, that is, they learn to ask for sponsorship ...Tibetans who do not 'adapt' to the way things work in exile express a fear of personal failure with coping in the new system altogether ... their young continually compete for the attention of aid organisations. To be connected with Westerners has become a kind of status in itself, despite the resentment of the foreignness it brings to the heart of the community.

Sponsorship and the support given to Tibetans by foreigners are, however, unstable and charged with ambiguity, and young people sometimes have to find more than one *rogram* in order to ensure a regular inflow of cash to survive. In the following section, I present and discuss the case of a young newcomer from Amdo and his struggles to obtain and conserve *rogram*.

Dorjee, a 26-year-old man from Amdo, had become extremely weak with malaria, and renounced his job in a McLeod Ganj restaurant. While staying in Delek Hospital, he had met one of the female interns and started a friendship with her. Before she left to go back to Europe, she promised she would ask her family to help, as she knew Dorjee's situation was desperate: with only one relative in the transit school and few friends at hand, he would not have much help after coming out of hospital. She was right: Dorjee's job fell through when he came out during the low tourist season, when the restaurant was not hiring any extra staff. His rent, which he shared with an Amdo monk for a small house with a leaky roof in McLeod, was 500 rupees a month. A few weeks after the young intern had returned home to Europe, he received 1,000 rupees from his new sponsor, the girl's father. Dorjee started to plan for the future, paid an upfront 300 rupees for a computer course, and set out on an Indian university correspondence course in 'social sciences', which I soon realised was due to my influence. The course booklets were in English and hardly accessible to Dorjee, who despaired of getting his qualification in time. His education had stopped after primary school, as his Chinese was not good enough to enter secondary education (he had been taught Tibetan grammar by a local kepo, or expert, in his hometown). His lack of an official end-of-study qualification stopped him from being able to access higher education and his Tibetan transit school leaver's certificate was not recognised by the Indian authorities. His only source of income had become his friend's father's *rogram*.

Three months passed, during which Dorjee received regular payments from his sponsor through the 'good bank' (the *ngulkang yagpo* or 'good bank', as he called the Western Union counter in McLeod) and his schedule had become that of a busy student. He enjoyed the classes but there was nothing to do in between, he said, only sitting at home and talking to friends about where to go next. Maybe Japan, maybe back to Tibet, he told me. He then decided to write to his sponsor saying that he would like to use the money to buy his own computer, which would allow him to study programming on his own. The irate Swedish doctor quickly replied that he was sending the money for Dorjee 'to do something with his life', and not to be wasted on computers. If he did not change his attitude, the Swedish man added, he would terminate the sponsorship. Dorjee told me that his sponsor had suddenly become very angry, and that he had sent a letter apologising but would not change his mind.

The prospect of losing the sponsorship did not seem to daunt Dorjee as much as I thought it would. Although he was reluctant to ask foreigners for help, he soon came to think of *rogram* as a natural gift from those much richer than him. In the small village on the road to Bagsu, Amdo youth gathered late at night to cook food and talk. Sharing food, clothes, books and money, the 'Amdo boys' discussed their fortunes. Dorjee explained that they sometimes slept very little because they stayed up late at night to discuss plans for the future. They often talked about returning to Tibet. Occasionally a member of the group would set out for the journey back, and for days Dorjee would be thinking of his friend, wondering if he should do the same. Those departures were accompanied by dramatic farewells, during which small gifts were exchanged and oral messages passed on for delivery back home.

The month after his argument with the sponsor, Dorjee lost his *rogram* and had to give up most of his classes. He could not find a job in Dharamsala and went to Majnukatilla in Delhi, where he secured work as a helper in an Amdo restaurant. Driven to depression because of the heat and inertia that reigned in the camp, Dorjee nevertheless stayed on in the hope of getting an Identity Certificate (IC) and finding someone who might help him get out of the country. After a month's waiting, he gave up on waiting for an IC and set out to help some friends selling dumplings in Bodh Gaya during the Kalachakra initiation. He often told me that he should have been more careful with the Swedish sponsor, and continued to ask around for English teachers, a common way to find sponsorship. When I offered to help after my return in England, Dorjee refused and said that my studies were more important, and that I would have no time to work. He said he would find another sponsor, even if this would take time, especially because, as a boy, it was difficult for him to gain the trust of potential *rogram* providers.

When I returned to Dharamsala in June 2002 and met Dorjee again, he had secured a permanent job in a restaurant where there was an abundance of foreigners who taught English (and therefore *rogram* opportunities) and free housing in a building adjacent to Namgyal monastery. He had discontinued his studies and made extra money by taking occasional trips to pilgrimage and teaching sites to sell handicrafts with friends. He planned for these trips on the basis of how much money he would earn at the restaurant, and the probability of making a significant profit from the outing. If economic necessity was not strong enough to compel him to go, he would stay in Dharamsala and spend time in the restaurant. He described his life as content, and told me he was getting used to being in Dharamsala. Rather than getting *rogram* for himself, which was too much trouble, he sometimes helped friends to obtain invitation letters or meet potential sponsors. He had, in a sense, become a *rogram* intermediary.

Dorjee's case is by no means archetypal, but provides a description of the kinds of motivations and concerns of young newcomers. Dorjee's position as a newcomer, and moreover as an older, uneducated man, excluded him from more institutionalised forms of sponsorship available to second- and third-generation Tibetans.

Yet the pervasive character of *rogram* had become a subject of concern among Indian residents and Tibetan elders, who saw it as symptomatic of social inertia, economic dependence and parasitism. This caused some acute tensions between the Indian and Tibetan communities. As one local Kashmiri trader told me:

> Some Tibetans, well most of the Tibetans are nice people. The ones who do business work really hard, especially the younger ones. But others just sit and wait for money, you know from sponsorship and other things. But you know, as long as the tourists come, then there will be sponsorship, so why should they work? And actually look, who would want to sponsor me? First of all, I am a Muslim, then, I do business, so people don't think I am poor. Then, I am Kashmiri, so sometimes they may think I am a terrorist [laughs]. So, really, nobody wants to sponsor me!*

In Dharamsala, newcomers and established families compete for *rogram* opportunities. For many families, *rogram* comes to supplement activities such as trading or working in the booming Dharamsala tourist industry. While earlier refugees used *rogram* for investment however, newcomers used it to procure everyday necessities: food, clothing, and medications. Inequalities were becoming more apparent.

Accusations and contagion

Newcomers are more likely to suffer from unemployment than older settlers, and also less likely to receive financial and social support from the extended social networks of the Tibetan diaspora. As a result, many are impoverished and likely to suffer from infectious diseases related to socio-economic deprivation, such as tuberculosis.

Young newcomers, many of whom had come to India specifically seeking employment or education, expressed concerns about their ability to achieve these goals in exile. Jamyang, a 25-year-old newcomer from Bompo (TAR), explains: 'This place is like a basket that is already full. There are already too many people here, and they already have jobs. If we want to work for the Tibetan government, they tell us our Tibetan is not good enough, can you imagine! If I cannot find work here I will have to go back to Tibet.'* This also has implications for health-seeking behaviour: 'I will not go to the hospital just to check my health, only for an emergency. I cannot afford medicines if there is something wrong with me, so I only go if it is free. Working in a restaurant, or making handicrafts you get almost nothing, you cannot save [money].'*

Many newcomers fall ill shortly after their arrival in India. Most commonly, illnesses are acquired in the so-called 'transit schools' where they are sent to gain language and practical skills. A visitor at the Soja 'transit' school near Dharamsala in 1998 vividly described newcomers:

> The newcomers are easy to spot. Their eyes are dull, their body language withdrawn. Often their cheeks are still raw from wind, sun and frostbite on treks from remote Tibetan villages that may take a month or more. The Tibetans call it the 'Transit Camp'. The Chinese, who are now aware of the 4-year-old institution, call it the 'Political Education School" ... At the Transit Camp they [the newcomers] are encouraged to return to Tibet to share their knowledge and to counter what Tibetans call Chinese propaganda against the Dalai Lama. Officials claim about 70% do.[5]

My visits to the transit school in 2000 and 2001 revealed that things hadn't changed much since this description, although efforts were being made to improve living conditions in the school. The barracks of the transit schools are a common ground for diseases like TB, malaria and dysentery. A leading Tibetan physician has described the burden of tuberculosis, in particular, as a 'humanitarian crisis': over 35,000 cases have been reported in the exile community since 1959. An epidemiological survey of TB incidence among Tibetans in India between 1994 and 1996 (Bhatia et al., 2002b) showed that groups with a substantial proportion of newcomers had all been severely affected by TB, for example students in the Doon Valley (14.8/1,000), the unemployed (23/1,000), and monks living in monasteries (17.2/1,000). The main referral centre for TB is Dharamsala's Delek Hospital, which applies the World Health Organization's guidelines for Directly Observed Treatment (Short Course) (DOTS) (Wares et al., 2000). This requires at least six months of uninterrupted directly observed treatment. Students, the unemployed, and seasonal traders are economically disadvantaged and highly mobile between settlements. They are therefore particularly vulnerable to diseases such as TB, less likely to be diagnosed, and less likely to comply with the immobilization required by DOTS.

In November 2000, I interviewed a Western physician working in Dharamsala's main TB clinic about her experience of working with TB sufferers. One of her main concerns was the non-compliance of TB patients who moved between clinics and took treatment 'breaks':

> For example, this girl [Tenzin] was found TB-positive in Bombay [Mumbai], then did not wait for her test results, went to Dehradun [Doon Valley, Uttaranchal] for more tests, did not wait again, and then went straight to Dharamsala where she was treated. She knew she was TB-positive and she took the risk of travelling all over the country! They expect the doctors to find solutions to everything, they take us for granted.*

What this physician characterised as irresponsible 'treatment tourism' had complex socio-economic roots. When I spoke to 20-year-old Tenzin on the TB ward, the other side of the story began to emerge: as a young student in a Mumbai technical college, she had run into financial trouble and taken up lodgings in a crowded student hostel. She also hinted that she had worked in bars as a 'hostess' to support herself, which suggested a possible involvement in commercial sex work. Tenzin knew that TB was common among Tibetan young people who travelled to Indian cities and decided to get tested soon after she felt the onset of symptoms. She became very apprehensive about the results after seeing one of her Tibetan friends quarantined in an Indian clinic with no relatives at hand for support. Tenzin decided not to wait for the results of her sputum test in Mumbai and returned to her 'home' settlement of Dehra Dun to seek her parents' advice. Her family were traders who travelled throughout India for the greater part of the winter season. Tenzin's parents were about to set off on their seasonal trip when she arrived, and therefore recommended that she go and seek competent care in Dharamsala's hospital. While she underwent treatment, friends and distant relatives were able to visit her and bring food to the ward. Tenzin stressed that she would not have been able to cope with the diagnosis or the treatment if she had been on her own in Mumbai:

> When you live in that city, you almost don't see any Tibetans. Many Indians think you are Chinese, or something else. When I was told I had TB and I had to stay there, I tried to call my family but they couldn't come here. I cannot go to college or to work wearing a mask, you know, then everyone will see that I have it. It's difficult … But if I don't wear a mask then maybe I give it to other people … I had to leave, to ask for Tibetan doctors' advice.

Tenzin's story reflects the complex influences on young Tibetans' lives: economic deprivation and social isolation contribute to shaping patients' health-seeking trajectories. For vulnerable groups, TB testing is a particularly momentous event: for traders, a TB diagnosis can mean the loss of the entire family's annual income; for students, an untimely diagnosis means being immobilised in a settlement where little social support is available.

Tibetan newcomers are easy targets for accusations of contagion. Earlier refugees tend to see newcomers as immigrants, and therefore as competition for jobs and sponsorship opportunities. In addition, newcomers bring echoes of home that often jar with second generation exiles' nostalgic imaginings of the 'homeland'. To many older settlers, newcomers appear rough and unsophisticated, incongruous in Dharamsala's cosmopolitan environment. In a process described by Sontag (1991) and Farmer (1993), the victims of disease are ascribed blame for contagion. In this climate of suspicion, rumours began circulating that newcomers were regularly sent from Tibet to 'spy' on activities in Dharamsala, in particular those of the government in exile. In a 1998 interview, Ama Adhe, a representative for the refugee reception centre in Dharamsala, explained:[6]

> Many Tibetan people who come from Tibet over to here are social parasites [in Tibet]. They are unemployed and they are culprits. They come over here saying that they have come into exile to receive the blessing of His Holiness [the Dalai Lama] but they simply don't have any good intentions. Then they say 'now we want to go back to Tibet' and when they go back they tell the Chinese that the Tibetan government in exile is bad and they tell the Tibetan people that the 'Tibetan Government in Exile does not care for us', they do not love us, they mistreat us as newcomers and spread rumors. Those rumors the Chinese like and the Chinese give them money and give them business opportunities in Tibet. This is what some newcomers do, but we do not have to worry about these sorts of people because they are only a small minority. They are beggars, thieves and robbers who are not even trusted back in Tibet.

Part of the problem, as identified by Adhe, obviously lay in the difficulty of separating 'good' and 'bad' newcomers. This was particularly difficult since 'bad' newcomers operated under cultural camouflage: 'They come here and their face is Tibetan and they eat and talk and do everything as every Tibetan. They are Tibetan by blood but they work for the Chinese. They have sold their soul because they get paid huge money.' The anxiety relating to newcomers is brought about by competition for already strained resources. Newcomers are therefore labelled as 'risk groups', with the tacit suggestion that they are putting others at risk. This is intrinsically linked to the idea that exiles are 'repositories' of true, 'authentic' Tibetan culture, and that newcomers are 'contaminating agents' both socially and physically.

These stigmatising discourses internal to the Tibetan diaspora had a visible impact on the groups concerned. For example, many newcomers became disillusioned because they did not find the community support they had wished for. One of my neighbours, who lost his wife to tuberculosis within the space of a few months, explained:

> We were both teachers, you see. We studied hard in Tibet, but we still had to go through transit school, even though we were teachers ourselves! My [Tibetan] grammar and my spelling is better than most people's, but … When my wife became ill, the doctor asked us how long we had spent in the transit school. He thought she had caught it there. She was not even supposed to go and she caught it there.

Another young male newcomer from Amdo said:

> People here think all newcomers have TB, that we are all sick, or taking drugs, or trying to, you know, do bad business. But it's not true … What I want is to work, I don't want to be ill! It's not our fault if we get ill here. In the monasteries it's even worse, because there are so many people sharing rooms, so many get ill.*

Newcomers' low socio-economic position makes them more vulnerable to diseases like TB, and more exposed to stigma. In addition, biomedical doctors from Delek described students of the newcomers' adult educational centre (Soja) as particularly prone to psychosomatic illnesses. These students were a major subject of concern for physicians, many of whom often expressed regret at not being able to visit the school more than once a week. Both the Mentsikhang and Delek doctors involved in the care for Soja students described their interaction with the students as very satisfying from both a professional and personal perspective. One Mentsikhang female doctor told me she felt extremely sad for the students. She could feel their own sadness and difficulties by the strong *lung* symptoms they manifested. She said: 'When I take the patient's pulse, usually it takes some time to find the personal pulse, then find the disorder, but with Soja patients, they have so much *lung*, it is the first thing you sense when you take their pulse.'

The school's barracks were a cluttered and closed environment of bunk beds, where intimacy could only be achieved by pulling blankets around one's bed, and space for personal belongings was kept to a minimum: a few boxes for clothes and objects were kept by the bed. In some of these impromptu cubicles were laminated pictures of family members and collages featuring poems or postcards from home. Two students showed me scrapbooks in which they kept diaries in Tibetan and Mandarin. One man displayed a picture of his girlfriend, a Tibetan teacher in Lhasa, in a staged photograph where she posed in a cinematic Chinese collar dress in a photographic studio. The boys' dormitories were ordered like army barracks but replete with souvenirs from home.

The school environment, adding to the trauma of exile and resettlement, can be considered a strong exacerbating factor in the development of psychological disorders and mental illnesses. Despite the fact that school residents have access to traditional Tibetan medicine, their first port of call for health-related matters is usually the local biomedical health worker. Students told me they did not have much time to speak with the doctors, whether Tibetan or foreign, because the physicians were on 'rounds' or 'just passing through'. They resented the scarcity of doctors' visits and the fact that it was so difficult for them to arrange a trip to Delek Hospital for serious health problems. At the transit school, biomedical doctors talked about the common discovery of a patient referring to 'pain in their neck, stiffness in the arms and the upper body'. One doctor explained: 'We could not diagnose any muscle stiffness, but it turned out that this patient has been tortured, and having dreams and disturbances, had lost his job and was unable to meet his family's needs. We see so many of these in Soja'. Here the psychosocial components of illness are clearly identified and related to the physical symptoms expressed by the student.

Both Delek Hospital and the Mentsikhang organise weekly visits to the Soja transit school. A Mentsikhang doctor sees approximately seventy to eighty patients a day during such visits. Physicians from Mentsikhang repeatedly told me that a great number of Soja patients had *lung* disorders, especially men. Newcomers and torture survivors are considered extremely susceptible to *lung* disorders. Traditional physicians were not the only ones to engage with the category of *lung*: most biomedical practitioners were aware of the importance of *lung* as a local idiom of distress and even directly questioned patients about *lung* disorders.

Politically informed notions of contagion and pollution are significant elements in exile conceptions of health and illness. Discrete social groups like newcomer refugees, by virtue of being associated with the danger of acculturation and social change, have become the focus of fears about social contamination. Thus the social boundaries that exiles set up amongst themselves are invoked in relation to disease to identify outsider groups as more 'at risk', more 'contagious', less 'socially responsible'. Such implicit moral allegations are intimately linked with the idea that earlier exiles are 'repositories' of true, 'authentic' Tibetan culture, and that outsiders, newcomers, and dissolute youths are 'contaminating agents' both socially and physically (Prost, 2004).

Conclusion – Part I

In the first part of this book, I have sought to show how exile impacts differentially upon the health of newcomers and older refugees. Many first-, second-, and third-generation exiles have developed strong social support networks. Newcomers, on the other hand, are often isolated and suffer a higher burden of infectious diseases such as TB. Their perception of the pathogenic effects of exile tends to centre around the threat of disease during their first few years in India and on the psychosocial adjustment to exile.

While exiles will 'shop around' for health-care, young Tibetans prefer to use biomedicine. Older Tibetans who suffer from chronic conditions, on the other hand, make extensive use of traditional Tibetan medicine. Tibetans from all generations and backgrounds use specific traditional prescriptions, such as *mani rilbu* and *rinchen rilbu*. These traditional medical preparations are tied to religious practices and to nationalist political agendas. Young newcomers have limited financial resources and may use traditional Tibetan medicine as a cheaper alternative to biomedicine.

Not only are newcomer Tibetans particularly vulnerable to illness, but they also have less social support to deal with bouts of ill-health and are more likely to be stigmatised for being 'infectious'. Exile therefore affects Tibetan refugees' health differentially: while more settled Tibetans may be able to mobilise financial and social resources to cope with illness in the family, newcomers are often marginalised and less able to deal with adverse events.

In the second part of this book, I examine the role of traditional Tibetan medicine as practised in Dharamsala's Mentsikhang and its contribution to public health in the Tibetan community. As highlighted in the first section, traditional Tibetan medical practitioners make a critical contribution to the care of Tibetan refugees within 'emic', local understandings of health and illness. Understanding how Tibetan refugees use traditional Tibetan medicine enables us to comprehend how exile has impacted on health in local terms.

Notes

1. As exemplified in the expression *'lus dang grib ma bzhin 'grogs pa'*, literally accompanying 'like a shadow', staying very close to someone.
2. 'mi'i ri mo nang la yod; stag kyi ri mo phyi la yod.'
3. 'spyi tshogs 'diy la nang mthongs gal chen po zhe drags red.'
4. These were coded in the following way: six newcomers (N), of which two were women (NF); four handicraft workers (H), of which two were women (HF), two male business owners (B), and three persons over fifty-five (G), of which two were women (GF).
5. World Tibet News. 1998. Dalai Lama encourages refugees to return to Tibet. Available online: http://www.tibet.ca/en/wtnarchive/1998/4/12_2.html (Accessed 24 July 2007)
6. Full interview transcript available from: http://www.rangzen.org/archive/98/06_india/adhe/ (accessed 24 July 2007).

Part II

The Role of Traditional Tibetan Medicine

Chapter 5
The Mentsikhang: Construing Traditional Authority

Counterfeit pills

In June 2000, an article entitled 'Counterfeit Pills' was published by the Tibetan Astro-Medical Institute (Mentsikhang) in Dharamsala. It warned of a crisis in the production of traditional Tibetan 'precious pills' (*rinchen rilbu*):

> Counterfeited Rinchen Rilbu (Precious Pills) are being sold by some unscrupulous people. In the public interest, we are sticking holograms of our logo on our packaging to distinguish our Rinchen Rilbu from the pretenders. If viewed in adequate light, our 3-D hologram depicts our registered logo with the word '*Mentsikhang*' inscribed in Tibetan & English. So, look for the shiny and silvery sticker on our Rinchen Rilbu.[1]

According to the Mentsikhang, the popularity of *rinchen rilbu* in India and internationally had spawned a trade in 'false' precious pills. The *rinchen rilbu*, small brown pills prescribed by Tibetan doctors as general vitality-enhancing medicines, contain a vast number of herbal and mineral ingredients. Their most 'potent' ingredient, however, is the blessings conferred on them by Buddhist lamas which 'empower' the medicines (*men drub*), giving them special potency. The Mentsikhang warned that counterfeit pills had not been blessed and were of lesser quality than their own.

The Mentsikhang is the 'official provider' of *rinchen rilbu* and of its simpler version, the *mani rilbu*. Both these pills play an important role in Tibetan exile health practices: the *mani rilbu* are small medicinal pills whose name derives from the fact that they are blessed through mantra recitations, or *mani*. They are collected by Tibetan families at the temple during religious gatherings and distributed to friends and relatives. The more expensive *rinchen rilbu* are often squirrelled away in drawers and brought out when an illness occurs in the family, or when someone needs an especially powerful blessing, before a trip abroad or a difficult exam, for example.

Both the *mani rilbu* and *rinchen rilbu* pills are important in the exile 'medicine cabinet', but the distribution of these pills in ritual gatherings gives them a broader, more complex significance. During religious meetings in the main temple (*tsuglakhang*), monks scoop the pills out of great jars and distribute them to the crowds assembled for prayers.[2] The practice of public *rilbu* distribution during temple meetings suggests that there is much more to exile public health than biomedical medicine. Ingesting *mani rilbu*, in itself a ritualised and innocuous act, is invested with a political significance specific to exile. The *mani* are commonly distributed during meetings and commemorations such as the Dalai Lama's birthday or 'Democracy Day', the anniversary of the Dalai Lama's endorsement of democracy for the Central Tibetan Administration. Temple gatherings use religious motives such as group prayers and ceremonies to galvanise political support for the Tibetan cause. In recent years, the Tibetan government in exile has fostered an explicit policy of support for traditional medicine. In 2003, for example, measures were taken to improve the health of young Tibetans through traditional medicine: 'In order to develop sound physical and mental health of [our] youth, the traditional health-care system relating to reproductive health and infant care have been re-introduced to the Tibetans. Mentseekhang reproduced special pills for the improvement of intelligence, which was distributed to all young children.'[3]

In the Tibetan exile communities, 'health' is imbued with strong religious and political overtones: in the official discourse, to safeguard one's health against the moral and physical perils of exile involves a commitment to both religious practice and political awareness. Tibetan 'precious pills' are charged with political meaning. For example, many exiles returning to the TAR and neighbouring Chinese counties carry with them pictures of the Dalai Lama (see Figure 5.1) and some of the blessed *rilbu* received at the temple. Tashi, a young Tibetan from Amdo who escaped to India and then returned to Tibet

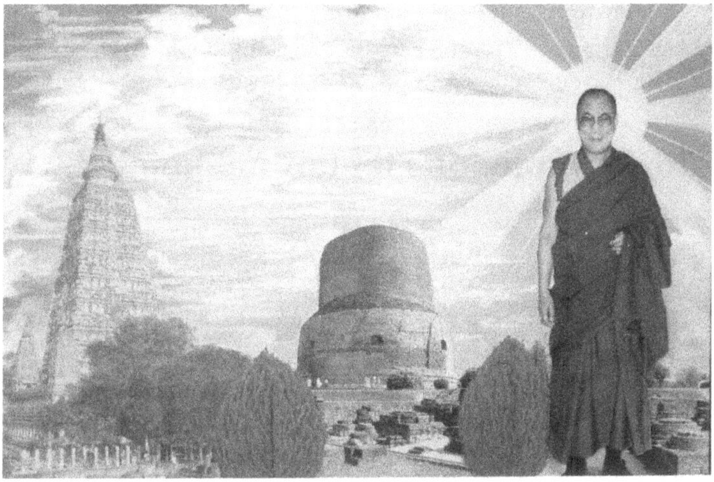

Figure 5.1: His Holiness the Dalai Lama with landmarks from Bodh Gaya. Such photographs can be found on street stalls in Dharamsala (Photo: Anonymous montage, 2001)

carrying political materials, told officials at the Tibetan Centre for Human Rights and Democracy:

> On my return to Tibet, I gathered around 32 booklets dealing with political themes, five audio cassettes containing speeches of the Dalai Lama and three documentary video cassettes containing footages on the invasion of Tibet which are all deemed political. ... I kept a small pack of *Mani Rilbu* (blessed pills of the Dalai Lama), a small portrait of the Dalai Lama and one booklet containing political themes. [...] I went to a rich trader's house and gave him some of the booklets and a small packet of *Mani Rilbu*. The trader refused the present and told me not to come again to his house as it might put him in trouble.[4]

The blessed *mani rilbu* are more than medicine: because they receive the blessing of lamas they are politically contentious. Exile health practices are inextricably linked to political agendas that promote public health as a matter of political allegiance to the Tibetan cause and to the Dalai Lama. The Mentsikhang has a critical role in producing these politicised medicines. This is not only the case in India, but also with the growing international clientele of Tibetan medicine, as the Mentsikhang's fight to defend its authentic *rinchen rilbu* demonstrates. In the following paragraphs, I offer a brief historiography of Tibetan medicine and look at the Indian Mentsikhang's current role in promoting health in greater detail.

Historiography of Tibetan medicine

Tibetan medicine has a long, rich, and complex history. Understanding the roots of Tibetan medicine is critical to analysing its contemporary role for Tibetan communities in exile.

The original transmission of Tibetan medical knowledge is attributed to Shakyamuni Buddha (the historical Buddha, who is thought to have lived in the 5th century BC). Shakyamuni is said to have given the first medical teachings to his Indian student Vimalagotra at the time of the first sermon (the turning of the wheel) in Sarnath (Meyer, 2002). In addition, further teachings were given in the Lotus Sutra, a text probably compiled in the first century AD and believed to be a discourse given by Shakyamuni toward the end of his life. The Lotus Sutra offers parables comparing the Dharma to a medicine and the Buddha himself to a physician.

The main Tibetan medical text, the *Gyushi*, is considered a *terma*, meaning a 'hidden treasure' or concealed teaching. As Gerke (2001) notes, in the Tibetan tradition the 'discovery' of such hidden teachings often corresponds to the historical date of the text's compilation. In fact, the actual origins and authorship of the *Gyushi* have been widely debated since the fourteenth century. While some authors argue that the text is a translation of an Indian Sanskrit work (Dash, 1986), others attribute it to the Tibetan twelfth-century physician Yuthog the Younger (Karmay, 1989). Emmerick (1977), on the other hand, contends that the present version of the *Gyushi* is based on Indian sources, mainly the *Astanga hridaya samhita*, a Sanskrit medical text written by Vagbhata and translated into Tibetan by Rinchen Zangpo. He speculates that the text must have been considerably edited and consolidated by Yuthog the Younger to reach its present form (Gerke, 1999). Increasingly however, authors agree that the physician Yuthog the Younger is the most likely author of the *Gyushi*.

The first known school of Tibetan medicine was founded under King Songtsen Ganpo in the seventh century AD, and was known as the 'Old Medical School'. Created by foreign physicians from China, India and Persia, the school focused on the translation of foreign works into Tibetan, and remained active until the eighth century. In the eighth century AD, Yuthog Yontan Gonpo the Elder, one of the nine court physicians of Tibetan king Trisong Detsen, started the 'New Medical School'. The eighth century is known as the reign of the Dharma kings because of the expansion of Buddhism promoted by three Tibetan rulers at that time. During this period, Tibetan medical literature and clinical skills were widely disseminated. This 'golden age' reached an end with King Langdarma (*ca.* 838–842), who is said to have destroyed the heritage of the Dharma kings along with the medical literature from that period.

In Western Tibet, however, the Tibetan medical tradition continued to flourish. In the eleventh century, Yesheod, King of the western kingdom of Guge, became the patron of the renowned Buddhist scholar and translator Rinchen Zangpo. Zangpo contributed to the development of a new medical school at Guge's main monastery, Tholing, by translating and editing Indian medical texts.

From the twelfth to the fifteenth century AD, the main medical tradition of central Tibet was the school of Yuthog Yontan Gonpo the Younger (*ca.* 1112–1203). However, other regions developed their own medical schools: while Western Tibet and Sakya evolved traditions that created their own texts and commentaries, other regions relied on oral sources and transmitted medical knowledge in family lineages. During the fifteenth century, however, the teaching of Tibetan medicine was split between two main medical lineages with different interpretations of the *Gyushi*. The first was based on the teachings of Changpa Namgyal Dragzang (*ca.* 1395–1475), and is known as the Changlug or Northern school, while the second was based on the teachings of Zurkharwa Nyamnyi Dorje (*ca.* 1439–75), and is known as the Zurlug or Southern school (Gerke, 1999).

The Tibetan medical curriculum reflects the intense knowledge exchange that took place within Tibet as well as with neighbouring countries from the eighth century onwards. Buddhism was not the sole cultural and spiritual influence to inform medical practice within Tibet: Bon, the indigenous religion of Tibet, was also a fundamental inspiration (Schrempf and Garret, 2003). The *Gyushi* itself is also a product of diverse influences and inputs: numerous commentaries have been added to medical curriculae over the years and are still studied as companions to the main text.[5] Finally, the transmission of medical knowledge through teacher–student lineages (*gyupa*) played an important part in shaping the curriculum and adjusting medical practice (Karmay, 1989; Meyer, 2002). The concepts and skills acquired by Tibetan physicians through their translation of foreign works as well as though the influence of teacher–student lineage traditions all contributed to the dynamism of the Tibetan medical tradition.

In the late seventeenth century, Desi Sangye Gyatso, minister to the Fifth Dalai Lama, synthesised the teaching of the Northern and Southern schools and founded new medical institutions (Parfionovitch et al., 1992; Gerke, 2001). The first was a medical school linked to the Lhasa government and located in Drepung monastery. Finally, in 1696, Desi Sangye Gyatso built the most important Tibetan medical college and hospital, the Chagpori ('Iron Mountain') medical college, which was named after the hill on which it stood in Lhasa. Gyatso also composed the most influential commentary on the *Gyushi* to date, the Blue Beryl (*Vaidûrya Ngonpo*), and had seventy-nine *thangka* paintings made to illustrate its contents (Gerke, 2001). Under the Lhasa government, Tibetan medicine became increasingly institutionalised: doctors were sent from Chagpori to the main provincial monasteries and districts to train new physicians. Others who trained in Lhasa set out to establish new medical institutions such as Yonghegong in Beijing (established in 1750), Kumbum (estab1ished in 1757 and now known as Ta'er monastery near Xining), and Labrang (established in 1784, now in Xiahe county, Gansu province) (Meyer, 2002).

At the time of the fifth Dalai Lama and Desi Sangye Gyatso, Tibetan medicine emerged as a state-sponsored system linked to dominant Buddhist sects. Tibetan medicine was, however, still practised in very diverse ways: while Mentsikhang-trained doctors maintained highly codified learning techniques, lay practitioners and diviners used a variety of practices, some of which derived from Bon beliefs, and continued to teach medicine through oral lineages. This 'division of labour' between different types of practitioners can be interpreted as a product of the complex tension between monastic

Buddhism and Tantric shamanic practices which characterised the rise of Buddhism in Tibet (Samuel, 1993).

In 1916, during the reign of the thirteenth Dalai Lama, the scholar and reformer Khyenrab Norbu founded the Lhasa Mentsikhang (Meyer, 2002).[6] The Mentsikhang diploma was a government-approved certificate. The college received one student from every major monastery in Tibet, thereby achieving unprecedented institutional control over the transmission of medical knowledge. Degree candidates memorised the *Gyushi*, and studied Tibetan grammar and poetry as well as anatomy and anthropometry (Meyer, 1992). Meanwhile, the thirteenth Dalai Lama strived to modernise health-care through the introduction of public health measures probably inspired by his visit to British India (Samuel, 2001: 262). In the final decades of the 19th century, biomedicine had made its entry into the Himalayan world through the import of missionaries and travellers, and through contact with representatives of British colonial rule in India (McKay, 2005).

In September 1951, soldiers from communist China entered Lhasa. In 1959, the Chagpori Medical College was destroyed during the bloody repression of Tibetans who had taken up arms against the Chinese. Some Tibetan physicians fled to India, others were imprisoned. In 1961, exiled Tibetan doctors founded a new Mentsikhang in Dharamsala. This new institution reclaimed the tradition of Yuthog the Younger as the inspiration for its own teachings. The first group of medical students from the Dharamsala Mentsikhang earned their degrees in 1966, followed closely by the first batch of astrology students in 1968. By the 1970s, there were seven doctors and six astrologers working at the institute. In 2002, the Mentsikhang had ten teachers and fifty-eight students.[7]

Since its inception in 1961, the Mentsikhang has trained over 200 doctors, the majority of whom now work in the institute's Indian branches. Access to Mentsikhang clinics expanded considerably in the 1980s, when twenty-one new sites were created, and then in the 1990s, with the creation of a further fourteen new clinics. The Mentsikhang now focuses a substantial part of its resources on research, with emphasis on the fields of cancer treatment, hypertension, and the alleviation of non-insulin-dependent diabetes mellitus (Namdul et al.,

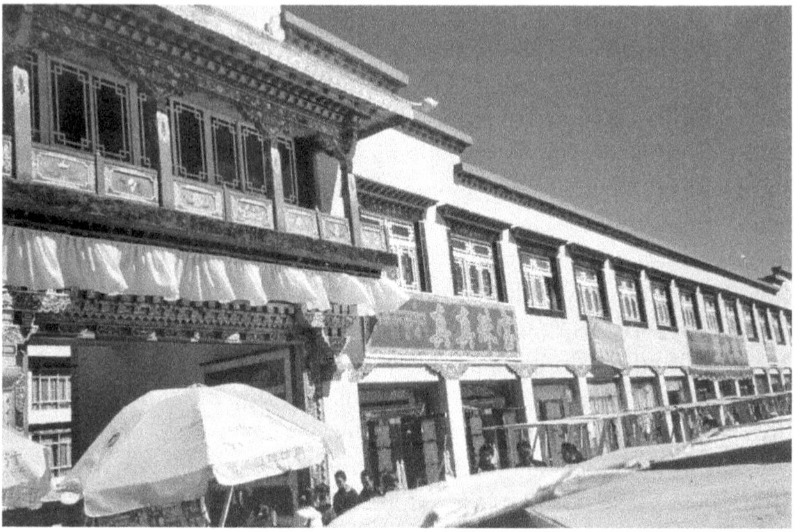

Figure 5.2: The Lhasa Mentsikhang in 2005. Physicians have offices on the two upper floors. The outpatient section is on the far right. (Photo: Murray Last, 2005)

2001). These projects have sought to legitimate the status of Tibetan medicine by proving its curative efficacy clinically through the use of Western clinical randomised control trials. Their stated aim is to enable Tibetan medicine to gain credibility vis-à-vis biomedicine and in the international scientific community at large.

Meanwhile, in Lhasa, the older Lhasa Mentsikhang has expanded, modernised, and become part of the Tibet Autonomous Region's public health system (Adams et al., 2005; see also Figure 5.2). Today, the 'two Mentsikhangs' have distinctly different identities but face similar problems: both are confronted to the commercialisation of traditional medicine and to the politics of 'legitimisation' via randomised controlled trials (Adams, 2002c). Both seek to find their place in complex and pluralistic medical fields, and both operate some degree of syncretism with biomedicine (Adams, 2002a, 2002b).

In the context of exile politics, medical practice has come heavily under the patronage of the Tibetan Government in Exile, and thereby tied to the Dalai Lama. The Mentsikhang's official title is 'Tibetan Governmental Astro-Medical Institute' (*bö shung menstikhang*), or sometimes 'Tibetan Medical and Astrological Institute of H.H. the Dalai Lama'. In the broader national and global context, Tibetan medicine has gained considerable renown, attracting both interest and criticism. Concurrently, Tibetan scholars are negotiating the terms of their relationship with biomedicine: clinical trials for various Tibetan medical products are under way, and frameworks for the 'legalisation' of Tibetan medicine are being discussed both in India and in the TAR. However, the politics of scientific legitimacy are very different in the context of the TAR and India. In the TAR, the Lhasa Mentsikhang is forcing an agenda of modernisation, attempting to prove the efficacy of an 'ancient tradition' through clinical trials (Adams, 2002c). This is partly driven by the commercial success of Tibetan medicine in the PRC. In exile, however, the defence of Tibetan medicine as a unique form of traditional Tibetan knowledge makes it a field invested with political significance and nationalist agendas, and this perhaps even more than any other form of exile 'cultural production', given its commercial potential.

Having charted some of the history of Tibetan medicine, the following sections describe learning processes and clinical encounters in the Mentsikhang in further detail. The aim of this section is to describe the contemporary practice of Tibetan medicine in Dharamsala's Mentsikhang and to highlight tensions between textual learning and clinical practice.

Learning, teaching, and clinical encounters in the Mentsikhang

Dharamsala's Mentsikhang clinic differs from its biomedical counterpart (Delek hospital) in several ways. Mentsikhang doctors usually receive patients in their own rooms or staff quarters rather than in a 'clinic room'. Doctors are put on a roster for consultations and rotate between the Mentsikhang's main building and the upper Mentsikhang clinic in McLeod. While most doctors will see about twenty patients a day, when visiting external sites they often see as many as eighty patients in an afternoon. Senior physicians have the opportunity to 'choose' their patients and are often given challenging or problematic cases. Senior religious figures have their 'personal' physicians in the Mentsikhang, but the majority of patients also return to see the same practitioners. The longest consultations generally last around twenty to thirty minutes. Tibetans sometimes visit with relatives and, as the consultation rooms are generally in private flats within the Mentsikhang compound, relatives are often invited to sit in. There are few 'physical incursions' on the body during a consultation and most patients remain dressed and seated in front of the practitioner.

In Dharamsala's Mentsikhang, pulse reading tends to be the preferred mode of diagnosis, and is more frequently used than tongue and urine analysis. For routine consultations, Tibetan doctors will 'feel' the pulse first and then rely on other diagnostic methods to complement this. Practitioners also check 'channels' (*tsa*) by pressing on various points on the body (for example on the back and neck). As part of the Mentsikhang requirements, the doctors jot down a list of observations in special notebooks. These notes summarise the observations and diagnosis made. Physicians also deliver a prescription for medicines (generally in the form of pills), which the patient can pick up at the pharmacy located on the ground floor of the institute.

Scholarly Tibetan medicine as practised in the Mentsikhang recognises roughly 404 gross types of diseases: 101 of these are considered incurable, 101 treatable with medical care, 101 self-curable, and another 101 due to *nopa*, harm caused by the intervention of supernatural beings (*lu*, water spirits, or *don*, demons) (Mentsikhang, 1995, 1998). 'New diseases', a category that would encompass cancers and Acquired Immunodeficiency Syndrome (AIDS), are often said to have arisen as by-products of modern lifestyles.

The *Gyushi* or Four Tantras enumerates three principal and four secondary causes of diseases. The three principal causes are: (1) lust, or desire, linked to the *lung* (wind) humour; (2) passion, or anger, linked to the *tripa* (bile) humour; and (3) dullness, or ignorance, linked to the *beygen* (phlegm) humour. The four secondary causes of illness are: (a) seasonal variations, cold and heat; (b) the action of an evil spirit; (c) the abuse of or mis-absorption of food; and (d) wrong behaviours and harmful lifestyles. The *Gyushi* lists appropriate dietary and behavioural rules to remain free from illness, taking into account different seasonal and astrological configurations. It enumerates the symptoms of disease and is a guidebook for the physician, listing questions to be asked in order to obtain information about the patient's diet, lifestyle and previous illnesses.[8]

In order to understand the dynamics of therapeutic choice and illness causation in the Tibetan exile community, it is important to understand the Buddhist framework that underpins medical practice and people's understandings of health. Therapeutic interventions and teachings on medicine are commonly introduced and concluded by injunctions to the eight Buddhas of medicine (*menla*). Preparatory ceremonies are carried out to increase the medical potency of substances and infuse them with the blessings of lamas. These are called 'empowerment' ceremonies (*men drub*). The *menla* are also called upon when students and doctors of medicine set out to collect plants, and when medicine is being prepared. The patients recite mantras of the Medicine Buddha (*Bhaisajyaguru*) when taking medicines and doctors also do so when undertaking therapeutic procedures.

The *Gyushi* classifies diseases in three categories: (1) diseases arising out of a humoral imbalance caused in this present life; (2) diseases arising from past negative actions, which are cured through religious practices and medicine; and (3) diseases arising from past negative actions, which are further aggravated by the patient's present condition.

This classification relates diseases to past actions in the sense that karma is thought to cause illness through the law of cause and effect (*gyute*). Tibetan medicine is deeply integrated with Buddhist practice and theory, which stresses the interdependence of mind, body and vitality. It traces the fundamental cause of all suffering to self-grasping or ego, which manifests itself in the form of *timug*, or delusion. This in turn gives rise to the three mental poisons: *dochag* (attachment, greed, desire), *shedang* (hatred, aggression) and *timug*. These three mental poisons will then cause 'imbalances' in the three humours: *lung*, *tripa*, and *beygen* (wind, bile, and phlegm). The *Gyushi* states that the bodies of elderly people are dominated by *lung*, those of adults by *tripa* and those of small children by *beygen*.

Since Tibetan medical aetiologies are related to Buddhist cosmology, patients often mention *le* (karma) as an explanation for disease. Doctors, in contrast, will rarely mention *le* during a consultation. Patients and doctors alike invoke *le* more readily in the context of diseases described in the Tibetan medical canon, and which can be treated by traditional Tibetan doctors, for example those due to imbalance of bodily humours or excessive consumption of certain types of foods. *Le* is less often offered as an explanation in the context of diseases with biomedical aetiologies. The argument that older and more religiously inclined patients favour *le* as a causal explanation does not always hold. For instance, when I questioned two India-born monks in their thirties on whether their *lung* and *beygen* imbalances (*beygen dang lung mugpo*) were caused by karma, they laughed at my suggestion and told me that not all things were necessarily related to *le*, but could also simply be *luki natsa*, or bodily disorders.

The *Gyushi* states that suffering is unavoidable and present from the time of birth, when the three poisons give rise to the physical body in the form of the three humours: wind, bile, and phlegm. Tibetan ethno-anatomy links the material to the spiritual: the five primary elements (earth, fire, water, air and space), which are the essential components giving rise, motion, and properties to all phenomena and consciousness, also give shape to the human body through the operation of a variety of winds at a subtle and coarse level (Meyer, 1992; Adams, 2004). The birth of a human form is contingent upon the presence of the regenerative fluids of a mother (red element) and father (white element), finding a home in a transmigrating consciousness (*sem*). The consciousness inherited from past lives meets with the five elements in the middle of the heart and rises as *sog*, the life force that gives shape to a human being. The type of body that results from this combination is dependent upon the type of wind that propels the consciousness and elements. The body of a human being that has not reached enlightenment is created when the *le ki lung* (literally 'the wind of karma), or karmic energy of negative past deeds 'disperses' the life force (*sog thu*).

The human body then develops around three main channels: *uma* (the central channel), *roma* (the right channel) and *kyangma* (the left channel). These channels and their forces intersect at key points or *khorlo* (Skt: *chakra*) within the body, and the movement of energies meeting and circulating at these points is described as 'circulating winds'. Other processes involved in the creation of a human body, complete with its white channels (created by the subtle winds) and seven bodily constituents (chyle, blood, flesh and muscle, fat, bone, marrow and reproductive fluid), are too complex to list here. However, a critical aspect in the formation and subsequent evolution of the human body is that the elements constituting it and those of the external world remain in constant interaction. Adams summarises this interaction beautifully:

> The body is never in a permanent state, always changing in relation to the climate, the seasons, the foods we eat, the emotions we feel in relation to our perceptions of the world around us, and even by the demonic or other harmful forces we come in contact with, and the karmic effects of action and intentions in past lives. (Adams, 2004: 288).

Buddhist theory and practice underpin Tibetan understandings of the body: Tibetan medicine, through its tantric roots, provides a link between the Dharma and the somatic system (Clifford, 1989). Tibetan ethno-anatomy encompasses a complex system of channels (*tsa tig*) and veins, where the 'subtle' physiology of humours is juxtaposed with the 'coarse' physical anatomy.[9]

Tibetans also have many terms to designate the body. The term *lu*, which designates the physical body, is commonly used in medical and religious texts. *Ku*, on the other hand, is a broader, honorific term referring to the body in relation to the world. It is also used in religious and medical contexts. *Sugpo* is the more mundane, non-honorific term that designates the individual body. All three terms lend themselves to complex metonymic associations. The term *ku*, for example, has manifold meanings: it can be used to refer to the physical body (*kusug*), or to a person (*kushog*, honorific), and is also commonly prefixed to names of parts of the body, thereby imparting an honorific connotation (Das, 1902: 88). *Ku* thus encompasses much more than simply the physical form of the body: it is also to describe a person's moral attributes, and other things pertaining to the body (e.g., *ku kam*, referring to a state of health and well-being). The diverse uses of *ku* reflect the links made by Tibetans between the body and the environment, but also between the body and the moral qualities of individuals. *Ku* is in this sense perhaps closer to the notion of 'person', than it is to that of 'body'. The word for longevity (*ku ring*), for instance, describes a quality pertaining to a person's physical *and* moral attributes. Hence one's 'bodily' well-being involves more than physical health, it engages the quality of one's relationships with others and with one's surroundings.

In the *Gyushi*, all disorders can generally be classified as hot, cold, or a combination of both. It is said that Tibetan medicine is particularly effective in the treatment of chronic conditions, such as arthritis, asthma, nervous disorders, and other conditions such as hypertension, hepatitis, coronary heart disease, bronchitis, and diabetes. This is also the view supported by Mentsikhang doctors, who claim that Tibetan medicine is more effective for chronic disorders and works over long periods of time, while biomedicine has more immediate but also more disruptive effects. One Mentsikhang doctor explained: 'Tibetan medicine and Western medicine are like two knives: Western medicine is sharp: it will cut off the finger and leave the root. Tibetan medicine is like a dull knife: it will not cut the finger off but work slowly to find the cause of disease.'

The allegorical tree depicting the root tantra of the *Gyushi* is often used to give a didactic explanation of the Tibetan medical system. Tibetan medical pedagogic *thangkas* depict medicine as a discipline with three major roots (*tsawa sum*): the root of aetiology, the root of diagnosis, and the root of therapeutics. The root of aetiology has two trunks: the first describes the body in 'dynamic equilibrium', the second the body in a diseased state. The body has seven constituents; when these are disturbed, it becomes diseased, as shown in the 'second root'. The third root, which is the root of therapeutics, has four trunks and describes the four methods of treatment in Tibetan medicine: diet, behaviour change, medicine, and accessory therapy. The root of diagnosis has three trunks: (1) visual examination (observation of tongue, urine); (2) pulse diagnosis; and (3) interrogation (*tiwa*), asking the patient about diet and lifestyle prior to disease.

Pulse diagnosis is a complex technique and is only mastered after years of learning and experience (Rabgay, 1994a). The physician places the index, middle, and third fingers on the radial artery in order to feel the patient's pulse. The three fingers exert different levels of pressure on the wrist. Each of the hand's three fingers is divided into an upper and lower division, totalling twelve divisions, and each division reads the pulse corresponding to a particular organ. The organs read by the index fingers are reversed when dealing with female patients. The physician checks a patient's pace and strength (or depth). It is said that a healthy pulse beats approximately five times within the completed respiratory cycle of a physician (*tsa len chig* being the Tibetan term for one beat of the pulse). Generally, if a pulse beats more than five times in one respiratory cycle, it indicates a hot disorder, whereas a pulse under five beats indicates a cold disorder. Variations in a healthy pulse are due to the difference in the natural, 'constitutional' pulses of individuals. The constitutional pulse is inherited from the influence of *le* (karma) as well as from parents' dietary and behavioural habits.

The most common form of treatment is herbal medicine (*tsa men*). The preparation of complex compound medicine can involve as many as eight types of ingredients: precious metals, soils, rocks, trees, resins, herbs, animals and juices. The quality and quantity of medicine administered is matched allopathically to oppose the characteristics of the disorder treated. Aside from herbal medicine, Tibetan doctors may use a number of mechanical devices to help them reach a diagnosis or cure a variety of ailments. For instance, different types of hammers (*tel*) (gold, silver, bronze and brass) are used in accessory therapy: the tip of the hammer is heated until it is red hot and applied on the disease point. These different types of hammers are used to treat cold disorders, excess accumulation of fluids in the joint, and conditions such as tumours or insanity. The golden hammer, in particular, is used to treat a lack of digestive heat, bodily aches, anxious mental states and epilepsy. While I have never seen such devices in consultations in Dharamsala, Mentsikhang doctors confirmed that they are still being used. Needles (*kab*), and specifically golden needles (*ser kab*), are used in the treatment of vertigo, dizziness due to hypertension, epilepsy, paralysis attacks, hysteria, insomnia and depression (these disease categories are the ones tentatively offered by Tibetan practitioners for Tibetan disorders). During my time in Dharamsala, I only heard one mention of a treatment with a golden needle, which was in the end refused by the patient, who thought it would be too invasive. Moxibustion, bloodletting and cupping are also sometimes practised to remedy a variety of disorders. These techniques are said to be used by doctors in the Mentsikhang, but I have rarely heard them mentioned and never seen them performed.

In practice, Mentsikhang doctors rely increasingly on herbal medicines rather than mechanical therapies. Furthermore, they are gradually phasing out the use of animal products in their medicines. In the early 1990s, visitors reported that animal products such as rhinoceros horns (ground for powder preparations) were still in use in the Mentsikhang, although such practices, illegal in India, are now banned. The secrecy surrounding the composition and fabrication of Tibetan medicines seems to have increased considerably since then, and it is now particularly difficult to have access to the formulations of preparations such as precious pills (*rinchen rilbu*).

The Mentsikhang's daily clinical work is shaped by prevalent health problems in the Tibetan population. Tibetans who spoke to me about their consultations at the institute were mostly middle-aged or elderly men and women suffering from chronic disorders such as stomach problems or hypertension. There is a strong emphasis on diet and the digestive process in the causation of disease, and doctors invariably give some form of dietary recommendations to their patients.

The Tibetan doctors' most common form of treatment is the prescription (*mentho*) of pills, generally two to three different kinds to be taken at set times during the day. Exiles are commonly seen taking such pills after a meal with a glass of boiled water. Traditional medical pills are usually sold for ten to forty rupees, a moderate cost for Tibetan exiles. They are cheaper than purchasing allopathic remedies (with or without subsidies) from the Delek pharmacy or from local chemists. As an example, a bottle of cough syrup will cost approximately ninety rupees in the pharmacies and fifty rupees at the Delek subsidised rate. Tibetan medicine can therefore be considered relatively inexpensive compared with biomedical treatments. Costly medicines such as *rinchen rilbu* (precious pills) are rare investments, and are often given and purchased as presents. The Mentsikhang also lowers or increases its prices according to patients' financial circumstances: poorer patients are likely to find their bills reduced by the pharmacy cashier, and some patients receive medicine free of charge (see also Samuel, 2001: 251).

In interviews, a number of Tibetans said: 'If Tibetan medicine doesn't improve your condition, at least it won't make you worse.' They often spoke of the duration of treatment (over months, sometimes years) as a testimony to the quality and mildness of Tibetan medical preparations. One elderly diabetic monk explained: 'Foreign medicine makes you better one time and then worse.'[10] Taking Tibetan medicine was thus seen as more advantageous because it would have no deleterious 'side effects'.

The next section explores the modalities of diagnosis and therapeutic choice through a case study of a young Tibetan monk afflicted by a *lung* disorder (see also Prost, 2006a).

Lobsang's *lung*

Lobsang entered monastic education at the age of nine and had a particularly successful ascent in the monastic hierarchy. He completed the degree of *Geshe*[11] at the young age of thirty and travelled widely as a member of the Dalai Lama's private office. A number of friends referred to him as a *mi chenpo*, an important person. Like many monks, he suffered from high blood pressure and had been told by both biomedical and traditional doctors to be mindful of his diet.

Lobsang's concern with health took a number of unexpected forms: he carried with him an electronic American sphygmomanometer and checked himself with it regularly. The instrument produced a strident noise once it had made its measurement, and was the subject of great admiration among other monks. This apparatus had earned him the nickname of modern monk (*kushog dengdu*), in reference to his fascination for Western luxuries and gadgets.

Lobsang did attempt to rein in his blood pressure by controlling his diet. On a number of occasions, he pointed out to me that diseases occasioned by high blood pressure were very common in the West among *mi chenpo*, men who assumed positions of power. This was due, he explained, to their high commitments and unnatural level of activity: high blood pressure was a disease of busy and important people. Now that Tibetans in exile had started enjoying some of the luxuries of the West, they also suffered its ailments.

Despite his efforts, however, Lobsang gained weight during my stay. He finally resolved to ask for the advice of an elderly and experienced Tibetan doctor from the Mentsikhang, who diagnosed him with a potentially dangerous form of *lung* imbalance.

Medical students had already explained to me that such *lung* illnesses are common in people involved in intellectual occupations, particularly in religious, meditative activities. *Lung* imbalances therefore characteristically affect monks and students of Buddhism, who, through their constant preoccupation with abstract considerations, sometimes become hot-tempered, nervous and irritable, as illustrated in the expression used for short-tempered people, *lung tsapo*, or literally: hot strong wind. Lobsang's particular illness arose from the overwork of his mental faculties, engrossed with spiritual matters. This had caused a dangerous increase of *lung*. Yet, even after the traditional doctor's diagnosis, Lobsang referred to his disorder as a 'BP' (blood pressure) problem, and was reluctant to engage with the traditional aetiology of *lung*.

The Tibetan herbal pills that Lobsang took punctually after every meal would be of no help to avert the danger of severe mental disorder. A urine diagnosis by his personal Tibetan doctor revealed large bluish-looking bubbles, confirming the diagnosis of a *lung* disorder. A radical treatment for this illness was to apply a long, heated golden needle to the cranium at prescribed points. Through this treatment, the symptoms of such a *lung* imbalance could be radically and permanently relieved. However, Lobsang was repelled by the invasive nature of this treatment, and persuaded his regular physician to let him continue his normal pill treatment. The doctor nevertheless asked him to go for a blood test at the hospital to check his sugar levels. Although Lobsang had heard his results in January, he only told me in April that they had suspected he had diabetes. The reason for his ambivalence in telling others about his suspected condition was, according to one of his relatives, linked to the fact that he did not want to be associated with other monks whose intake of rich foods was thought to have triggered their diabetic condition.

Lobsang thus avoided the local hospital, where nurses could gossip about their patients' illnesses, and retreated to the quiet haven of the Mentsikhang. The diagnosis and rapid treatment of diabetes have become a public health priority in the Tibetan community. One possible traditional form of treatment consists of a daily half cup of bitter gourd juice and blackberries in black dhal with a spoonful of honey. The roots of blackberries are traditionally used in Ayurveda to treat diabetes, and the bitter gourd's essential property is to reduce the level of sugar in the blood. When I asked Lobsang whether he believed this illness might have been caused in some way by karma, he said: 'If that is the case, then everything is caused by karma.'

According to the traditional Tibetan doctor who had treated him, Lobsang's busy lifestyle, rich diet, and high level of intellectual activity had caused the imbalance. Behind this diagnosis lurked a slight reproof of the Geshe's quick social ascent in the exile religious hierarchy. The choice of golden needle treatment implied that there was a serious *lung* problem to be treated.[12]

Tibetan exiles are meaningfully selective in the way they present and legitimate the intervention of environmental factors, humours, karma, and the relationship between these factors in the course of their illnesses (Prost, 2006a). Some will relate the emergence of disease to personal histories and karma, physical and social constraints, and the hardships of exile. Others yet, such as Lobsang, sideline karmic explanations in favour of causation narratives focusing on biological aetiologies. Geshe Lobsang's reluctance to adhere to a karmic explanation, and his choice to segregate the biophysical from the social, are a reflection of his concern with social status and exile politics.

Lobsang is of course not unique is using causation narratives to legitimise his social position. In the daily practice of medical choice-making involving the elaboration of complex explanatory models for illness, exile Tibetans operate negotiations between a traditionalist view allocating the causes of illness and misfortune to karma, and therapeutic choices dictated by social circumstances. Karma is a concept that can give meaning to traumatic events, but it can also be a means of avoiding questions and potential criticism (the explanation 'it was karma' can then act as a 'silencing' statement, fending off further questioning). As such, it can be seen as a contextual 'tool' rather than an ontological statement.[13]

The experience of being ill connects the embodied experience of exile (the constant maladjustment and discomfort of the body in exile surroundings), with subjective interpretations of illness and misfortune constructed out of individual biographies. Some disorders, such as *lung* imbalances, have emerged as specific problems linked to the hardships of exile. The physical environment of exile further exacerbates such disorders: *lung* imbalances occur primarily in the hot summer season, when Tibetan refugees recurrently complain of the heat in the Indian settlements (some told me that they saw religious teachings coinciding with the monsoon as an opportunity to clear the accumulation of *lung* built up during the summer).

In the context of the TAR, Adams and Janes have described *lung* disorders as a somatised 'weapon of the weak', a syndrome through which Tibetans articulate individual experiences of oppression and resistance. Connor finds that the role of Tibetan medicine is then to provide 'a context in which people can express their distress in their own cultural idioms as a vulnerable and disenfranchised minority in the People's Republic of China, subjected to forms of racism' (Connor, 2001: 16). From this perspective, *lung* designates a force operating both inside the body as a humour, but also outside the body as a social and moral force. *Lung* links the social and the political by encompassing 'the political as part of bodily suffering, and as [an] expression of the social and moral connections between people' (Adams, 1998: 92). Adams and others have suggested that the Tibetan body is partly constituted by the social, and experienced at least to some degree as a 'collective' body. Indeed, phenomena such as '*lung* epidemics' manifest the suffering of individual Tibetans as one 'body politic', in Scheper-Hughes and Lock's terms (1987).

In exile, dealing with prevalent disorders such as *lung* imbalances has become a matter of 'public health'. In order to survive and prosper, Tibetans must address the social and economic problems in the settlements, some of which are embodied by *lung* sufferers like newcomers. Because Tibetan medicine places emphasis on the interrelatedness of environmental, social, and moral determinants of health, it is particularly suited to addressing conditions caused by the move to exile and long-term adjustment. In the next chapter, I examine recent changes in the teaching and practice of Tibetan medicine within Dharamsala's Mentsikhang.

Notes

1. The note of caution is still 'up': see http://www.Mentsikhang.org/caution/ (accessed 6 February 2005).
2. The *mani rilbu* distributed at the temple are wrapped in paper bearing the notice: '*Thig chen chos gling tsug lag khang du 'gong sa 'skyabs mgon chen po dbu bshugs kyis ma ni dung sgrub mdzad pa'i rten 'dus ma ni ril bu,*' explaining that the *rilbu* were blessed by one million *mani* or mantra recitations in the temple.
3. *Tibetan Bulletin*, 2003, 7(4): 3.
4. Tibetan Centre for Democracy and Human Rights monthly update, May 2002.
5. The most famous commentaries are the 'Oral Instruction of the Ancestor' (*Mes po'i zhal lung*) by Zurkha Lodo Gyalpo (1509–179), Desi Sangye Gyatso's 'Blue Lapis Lazuli' (*Baidurya sngon po*) and 'Amplifications' (*Lhan thabs*) (Gerke, 2001).
6. The Dharamsala and Lhasa 'Mentsikhang' have the same name. However, the spelling most commonly used for the exile institute is 'Men-tsee-khang', while the Lhasa school is usually referred to as 'Mentsikhang'. (Karmay, 1989: 20; Gerke, 2001: 31).
7. Astrology suffered a considerable decline at that time and the majority of students were taking the medical degree (*sman pa ka chu pa*).
8. Meyer, 1992; Clark, 1995.
9. Actual veins are supplemented by 'subtle veins', in which the bile humour (*beygen*) operates, supporting the Nirmanakaya, or form body. Subtle airs activate the *mkhris pa* humour, which generates the Sambhogakaya, or apparitional body. Subtle essences vehicle *rlung* and animate the Dharmakaya, the ultimate truth body.
10. '*rgya sman phyog gcig nas phan kyi yod red a ni phyog gcig nas gnod kyi yog red.*'
11. *dge bshes*, or the equivalent of Doctor of Philosophy in the Tibetan monastic system.
12. The humour *rlung*, generally translated as wind, is one of the three fundamental forces that regulate the functioning of the body. It is traditionally said that the mind rides on *rlung* like a horseman on his mount, illustrating that this humour is akin to a nervous system, largely responsible for carrying and regulating emotions and states of mind. An imbalance in *rlung* can have grave consequences for the mind: a block in the healthy circulation of *rlung* can lead to mental sickness and even insanity.
13. This is congruent with Janes's findings in the TAR: 'Interviews with a wide variety of Tibetans from different backgrounds show that they express notions of causality that mix notions of mind management, appropriate social behaviour of self and others, pollution or defilement, the actions of deities and demonic misfortune, misfortune or bad luck, strong or poisonous emotion, diet, and weather' (Janes, 1995: 11).

Chapter 6

Humours on Trial: The Mentsikhang's Dilemmas

A business unlike any other

A few yards down the road from Dharamsala's Tibetan Delek Hospital, an imposing metal gate opens onto a labyrinthine complex at the heart of Gangkyi. A strong aroma of dried plants and the characteristic odour of burning juniper leaves (*shugpa*) diffuse through the Mentsikhang courtyard. The compound looks deserted at first, with only a few children chasing bicycle wheels in the dust. The soft rumble of large copper pill makers is heard in the distance. Looking up to the quarters where staff live and hold their consultations however, one soon becomes aware of a quiet buzz of activity. Patients disappear behind door curtains, while others make for the pharmacy office with prescription notes. Students, their afternoon lectures completed, wander out to the local shops and restaurants in Lower Dharamsala.

My first dealings with the Mentsikhang and its doctors were difficult. My interest, as I explained to the Mentsikhang director who granted me an initial interview, lay in the functioning of the institution itself: I wanted to know how much medicine Mentsikhang produced, of what kind, and what percentage of it was exported. The director's response was firm:

> You say you want to look at statistics, production. We are not a business, we do not want to be big. If you look at the way we run the institution, you will see that costs equal profits. We sell at the cost of raw materials. What costs one rupee here will cost $100 in the US because retailer, wholesaler and distributor all get a share.*

> We are not in our country, we have to protect ourselves. It is because of the protection of His Holiness and the greatness of the Government of India that we can do this. We are competing with Ayurvedic medicine and biomedicine. We do not want to go through legal procedures in Europe and the States. It takes 20 years to be recognised as a medical system. You have to do tests. What does it mean? Tibetan medicine is more than a thousand years old, we don't need this. If you are going to give a Tibetan pill to a rat and wait, watch for it to suffer, and then try another and another, this will not work.

Our discussion continued into a conversation about the 'proper way' to study Tibetan medicine. Rather than studying the Mentsikhang's 'modern' dilemmas, I was told to learn about the practice of Tibetan medicine itself:

> If you want to learn about Tibetan medicine, then you have to go to the root, learn about the history, the peripherals. There are three elements in Tibetan medicine (*lung*, the wind that goes through the body, the liquid in the body, phlegm, *beygen*, and bile, *tripa*). With these three you have everything.
>
> Do you believe in the soul? We Tibetans believe in the soul but when you look for it, it is difficult to find it. You will find that more old people like Tibetan medicine, the young want quick relief. Tibetan medicine has a long-term effect. His Holiness says: 'Tibetan medicine works best when you are not ill.' It helps maintain a balance between healthy body and mind.
>
> There are three methods. First diagnosis: check the eye, tongue, pulse and urine. Second: prescription, it is not the same for every category [of disease]. When a disease is not very serious, the doctor asks patients to change [their] habits, drink and food. If it is more serious, then the patient should change his habits and take medicine. If it is very serious then you can have treatment like moxibustion or gold needle.
>
> Many VIP media people come here and say, 'Ah, you diagnosed my disease, I have been doing this and that treatment for years but no one had diagnosed my disease right.' Not many people are open about it, but some are. Here it is considered medicine; in the US it is food supplement! Go to the root, study the peripherals, then look at numbers and then write your book.*

The director had listed the main qualities traditionally attributed to Tibetan medicine: holism and diagnostic accuracy. The discussion had also unveiled some preoccupations about the Tibetan medicine's relationship with biomedicine and other medical systems, and, more specifically, about the Mentsikhang's legal status. From the point of view of this senior and respected administrator, this was indeed a turning point in the Mentsikhang's institutional life.[1]

Creating institutional identity

In a study on the institutionalisation of Tibetan medicine conducted in the Tibetan Autonomous Region (TAR) from 1988 to 1993, Janes stated that:

> In the expansion into the state bureaucracy, Tibetan medicine has acceded to institutional modernity through transformations in theory, practice, and methods for training physicians. With the collapse of the traditionally pluralistic Tibetan health systems into the professional sector of Tibetan medicine, contemporary Tibetan medicine has become to the laity a font of ethnic revitalisation and resistance to the modernisation policies of the Chinese State. (Janes 1995: 6)

In exile too, Tibetan medicine constitutes a fund for ethnic revitalisation: it is part of the portfolio of 'authentic' Tibetan practices to be preserved for future generations. During the course of fieldwork, I was often told that students and doctors at the Mentsikhang were upholders of a traditional and internationally recognised knowledge recognisable as uniquely Tibetan. The length and depth of traditional medical training are considerable: five years for medicine and astrology respectively, comprising teachings on grammar, versification, Buddhism and botany. The study of Tibetan medicine is reputedly so difficult that only the most gifted students succeed in the entrance examinations (*yig tse*), and, later on, in the yearly tests. Most Mentsikhang students have been educated up to the twelfth grade and must have a very good proficiency in Tibetan language to pass the examinations. This is a significant obstacle for students from Ladakh or Nepal, many of whom have little or no education in classical Tibetan. Students admitted to the Mentsikhang are therefore considered to be among the most gifted young Tibetans in exile. After the set five years and a year's worth of work experience (*nyamtog*),[2] the Institute guarantees the students employment in one of the Mentsikhang's branches in India or Nepal. One female first-year student comments:

> It's not that I always wanted to study Tibetan medicine. But I was very good at grammar and Tibetan language at school, and my uncle is a well-known doctor in the Mentsikhang. I thought this would be a good profession, where you do good for people, especially here, where people have so many problems. And then I knew I would get work straight after. Many people when they come out of TCV, they don't know what to do, they have to go and look for foreign sponsors to go and study or go to Delhi or something. Here I don't have to do that. I have a sponsor for my studies but I know I will be able to work after that.*

The Mentsikhang precinct is similar to a small campus. Students share dormitories and take their meals together in a refectory at set times in the morning and evening, taking turns to cook for each other. The students are geographically and hierarchically separated from the staff, whose quarters are in separate buildings. However, almost all members of staff, from pharmacy workers to students and teachers, live within the constantly expanding Mentsikhang compound. This is partly due to convenience, and partly because of the financial incentive of subsidised or free housing. Mentsikhang staff have a strong sense of identity and attachment to the institution, as explained by a pharmacy worker:

> Since I arrived at the Mentsikhang, I've always lived here. We know all the doctors and astrologers. We have family here, so, if someone needs help with children, we always have friends or family to look after children… I feel very proud to work at the Mentsikhang, it is a very important place. You are always learning a lot, and the work generates merit.

To outsiders, Mentsikhang students form an integrated, cohesive group, organising their own activities and social life. They regularly put on events such as plays and fairs, which government workers and nearby residents are invited to attend. Although such institutional participation in cultural events is by no means exceptional in Dharamsala, the Mentsikhang students have a reputation for putting on some of the best song and dance performances (*lugar*) in the settlement. Indeed, one may think of students' training at the Mentsikhang as an 'institutional apprenticeship' (Freidson, 1970; Sinclair, 1997). The Mentsikhang is a bounded space, a form of 'total institution': many of the students do not leave their training location but live and practise medicine within it. One female physician who had recently graduated from Mentsikhang said:

> I met my husband while studying at the Mentsikhang, and his grandmother lives here with us, to look after our son. If I am not able to see a patient, I can send my husband, and he will do the same thing ... Yes, we are often invited to government events, like the birthday of His Holiness and other things, then we go as a group, with other doctors from Mentsikhang.

Learning medicine at Mentsikhang

In addition to its institutional identity, the Mentsikhang has also created an exclusive 'cognitive identity', focused on textual learning, recitation (*katon don*) and examination.[3] Within Tibetan exile society, the institution that most resembles the Mentsikhang is the monastery. In many respects, medical training follows a pattern similar to religious training, with a similar emphasis on rote learning, recitation and repetitive examinations. Students in the monastery and the Mentsikhang are educated according to the same pattern: first, they memorise key texts (in the Mentsikhang, the *Gyushi*); secondly, they listen to explanations of these texts and learn about the main commentaries; and, finally, they debate the content of the texts with each other. At the end of their training, medical students undergo examinations in the form of question and answer sessions reminiscent of the monasteries' debating exercises. As Millard asserts: 'Education in medical school is consonant with the wider cultural pattern of Tibetan education' (2002: 85). One older monk and physician explained how his monastic training had helped him study medicine:

> Reciting texts is easier for me, because I have practice from the monastery. At the Mentsikhang we have to learn the *Gyushi*, but also to recite other texts which list many parts of the body. For example, we have to learn all the channels in the arms, and the name of the different pulses! But to know something by heart means you never forget it.

Training at the Mentsikhang involves undertaking a number of Buddhist practices, many of which are also taught in monasteries. At the start of lectures (*katam*), students recite verses requesting the teachings of the Medicine Buddha (*Bhaisajyaguru*), as well as the Medicine Buddha's own mantra. During lectures, students learn about the eightfold way of medical practice (*menla yanglag gyepa*), an echo of the eightfold path of Buddhist practice taught in monasteries. When prescribing medicines for particular conditions, a physician is thought to act as an intermediary between the patient and the divine: the person taking medicine has shared the blessing of the deity with the lama and is bound by a vow (*damtsig*), which enforces the bond between patient, healer and deity. Breaking the vow is seen as a potential source of illness (Clifford, 1989: 68).

The most advanced spiritual practice undertaken by physicians is perhaps that of meditating on the medicine mandala. The mandala has three levels of interpretation and realisation. First, the physician identifies with the Medicine Buddha; this constitutes the 'inner level'. Then, the practitioner identifies her own body with the medicine mandala (the secret level). Finally, the physician professes and practises devotion to the Buddha and medicine (the external level). The mandala can be meditated upon in its material form (as a sand mandala or *thangka*), visualised, or 'realised' through the tantric practice of identifying one's body with the mandala.[4] I asked the physician monk quoted previously in this section whether the practice of meditating on the medicine mandala was still carried out today:

> **Physician:** All doctors make offerings and dedications to the Medicine Buddha. But to identify one's body with the medicine mandala is something that not many people can do.
> **AP:** What teaching do you have to receive to be able to do that?
> **Physician:** Some of my old teachers [from Tibet] knew how to do it so they taught me, but I only teach those who want to know. Many doctors now feel this is not necessary for their patients.

The religious component of medical training is also manifest in physicians' subsequent practice: they perform recitation of mantras during certain forms of treatment, such as moxibustion (*metsa*) or golden needle therapy (*ser kab*). They are also meant to perform a dedication of merit to the Medicine Buddha before consulting with a patient, although in practice, time constraints mean that this is seldom observed. Many also undertake personal pilgrimages to holy Buddhist sites in India (see Figure 6.1).

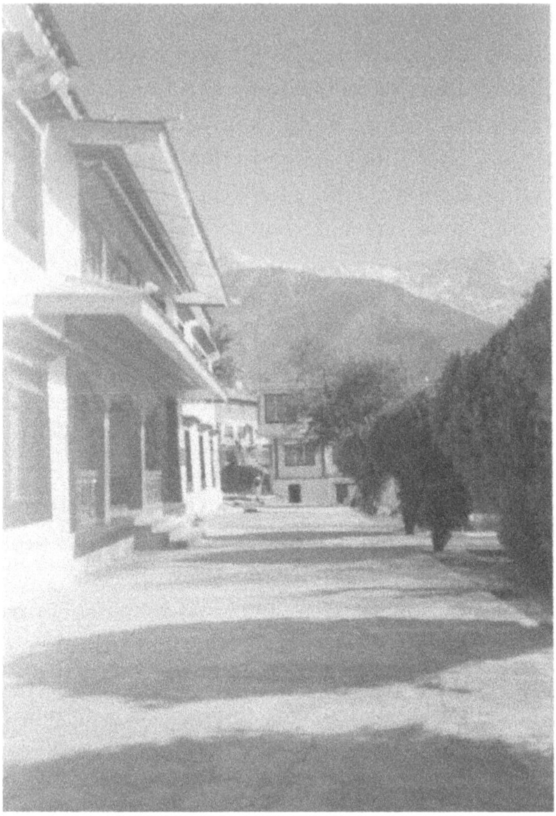

Figure 6.1: Library of Tibetan Works and Archives (Dharamsala, Himachal Pradesh). (Photo: Audrey Prost, 2001)

One student drew an interesting parallel between learning medicine and learning *chö*: 'We are told that if you know the root tantra of the *Gyushi* (*tsa gyu*), you know the essence of medical knowledge; this is like saying that if you master the *prajna paramita* [the diamond sutra, a famously complex Buddhist text], you know all there is to know about Dharma.' Therefore, if one masters the *tsa gyu* in all its complexity, one has mastered the essence of medical teachings.

It is also important for students to be literate in Tibetan language and grammar, and to master the complexity of medical terminology.

For this purpose students use mnemonic devices derived from religious training (mostly lists and versification) in order to memorise the names of physical organs, their attributes and the properties of medicines. This practice of memorising 'lists within lists' is also commonly used in monasteries when learning Buddhist texts. In practice, the student must be able to go through the roots and branches of the allegorical tree of medicine, including its roots, trunks, branches, leaves, flowers and fruits and to 'unfold' them as lists of procedures, diseases and treatments. In the context of a consultation, a physician can unfold the lists backward from specific symptoms (e.g., dizziness) to general aetiologies (*lung*), or forward, from the general (for example, finding that the patient's body is dominated by the humour *bey gen*) to the particular (the need to recommend specific types of food). An older female physician explained:

> The trees are like indexes. You can go through the tree, through the root, the branches, the leaves, and then you are able to find what particular symptoms this disease has and also at the same time to know what is its cause. So it helps you to have a better vision.*

The versification of medical texts into nine syllable phrases (*tsigkang*) for easy memorisation also seems to be inherited from religious teachings. Many students make taped recordings of recitations of the *Gyushi*, which they can then listen to in their spare time to facilitate memorisation. I was told that one particular recording of the *Gyushi* made by a monk medical student was particularly valuable because he had the perfect 'pitch' and 'pace' of recitation, a skill he had gained after chanting and reciting texts in the monastery. Students also commented that monks have a facility for medical training due to their trained powers of memorisation.

Finally, students are told to treat medical teachings as those of the Medicine Buddha himself, to focus their religious activity on him, and to handle medical texts as they would religious ones (by placing them on their head as a sign of reverence for instance). Many of the Mentsikhang's learning methods therefore derive from religious training.

Behind the scenes

In less formal learning settings, there is considerable cooperation among Mentsikhang students. They feel each other's pulses, learn the preparation of medicines from each other, and go on annual plant collecting trips together.[5] They also regularly help each other to memorise texts by going through thirty-minute question and answer sessions, or making each other recite sections of the *Gyushi* in mock examinations.

Most students confess a tendency to idealism, and view traditional medicine as a merit-generating occupation in both a religious and political sense: medicine generates good karma, and is a practical way of helping fellow exiles, as a senior Mentsikhang teacher explained:

> There are people who meditate, like monks and nuns. This is very good. There are people who travel, speak about Tibet and Tibetan freedom, like His Holiness [the Dalai Lama]. This is also very good. Then there are physicians like us. We see people suffering everyday, Tibetan exiles, and we can do something. It is a small thing, but it helps. Also there is pride in the fact that this knowledge is Tibetan, it comes from the past, it comes from the Medicine Buddha, but it is used to solve contemporary [*dengdu*] problems.

Although the profession of Tibetan traditional physician is enviable because of the status it affords, it is certainly not the most lucrative job in exile and salaries are lower than those offered at the biomedical hospital. Furthermore, students know that they are likely to be sent to 'difficult' placements in other parts of India, where working conditions can be difficult. Yet one enthusiastic young male student explained: 'I am not there to earn money, but merit is worth more than money, you can take it in your next life!'

Doctors who have concluded their year of professional experience (*nyamtog*) and come back to the Mentsikhang will characterise their time in other branch clinics as an opportunity to 'work for the community', or 'giving something back'. Students jokingly refer to these placements as the '*bardo*', or the passage between death and rebirth in Tibetan Buddhism.

Medical knowledge is transmitted with a step-by-step progression through the tantras, culminating in the final year's teaching of the

Gyushi's Final Tantra (*chima gyu*). Examinations are conducted at the end of each year. In the final examinations, students have to diagnose a set number of patients' diseases correctly (usually forty), and must undergo four hours of text recitations examined by their teachers. Students described this final test has a gruelling and climactic moment.

The normal learning schedule consists of four hours of lectures from 9 a.m. to 1 p.m., and free afternoons for 'self study', during which students learn texts. Students usually get up around 7:30 a.m., and then sing the Tibetan anthem before classes begin at 9:00 a.m. In 2000, two hours each week were devoted to classes in 'Western' science, including anatomy and physiology. Students are expected to contribute small articles in English to the college journal *gang ri la tso*. In this journal, they often debate similarities and differences between biomedical and Tibetan ways of treating diseases, as well as the health hazards of exile modernity, such as smoking or unhealthy lifestyles. Students are also required to give public presentations, which are meant to hone their public speaking skills. Some of the students I interviewed also used their free time to study biomedicine through biology books purchased in local Indian stores.

According to some Mentsikhang students, the increasing emphasis on 'Western science' in the curriculum has been brought about by patients' new expectations of Tibetan physicians. This was described as a recent development. As a young Tibet-born male student put it:

> In Tibet, and still now with most Tibetans, when someone goes to see a doctor, and the doctors says 'Eat this food, do not eat this food, eat this medicine', they just say 'Fine' and do as the doctor says. These days, some of these foreign people, they come, and they go and they see a doctor, then they ask lots of questions: they want to know what the medicine is, how it is made, what exactly the disease is. Then it becomes very difficult.*

Another student who had been listening to this conversation joined in:

> Yes, then there are patients who are bad mouths [*gyagka*, or literally 'shit-mouthed'] … evil-minded [*ngan sempa*] [laughs]. There are two types. Some have a bad mind [*sem nagpo*]. They come to the doctor when they are not ill, and, when the doctor just tells them they are healthy, get angry and refuse to take advice, saying the doctor is bad

> and does not know enough. This is one type. The second type is [when] some patients do not want to listen to the doctor's advice and just carry on doing as before, then come and complain that the medicine did not make them better.

Students described instances when patients would go to Delek Hospital and then come to Mentsikhang with their diagnosis and prescription to ask 'what else' could be done. In such situations, they said, it was important for physicians to understand the meaning of the biomedical diagnosis and the nature of the tests that had been conducted.

Student responsibility in patient treatment is extremely limited (although students do practise pulse reading on each other and this is considered *nyamti*, or 'teaching through personal experience'). During the five-year training, there is almost no clinical practice. Experience is generally gained during the student's one-year placement with a Mentsikhang branch after the completion of the diploma.

The following section looks at the curriculum of the Mentsikhang and at recent changes in teaching.

The curriculum: studying the *Gyushi* selectively

After studying for five years to earn the degree of *Menpa kachupa*, Mentsikhang graduates undertake one to two years of clinical experience under the supervision of a qualified physician in one of the school's forty-three clinics. Their education is divided into five semesters with breaks for the Tibetan New Year (*losar*) and plant collecting trips. The curriculum given to me by the teachers and published by the Mentsikhang in 2002 mainly focuses on the study of the *Gyushi*. The compendium is composed of four tantras, which are studied one after the other:

1. The Root Tantra (*tsa gyu*)
2. Explanatory Tantra (*she gyu*)
3. Oral Instruction Tantra (also called Quintessential Tantra or *men nga gyu*)
4. Subsequent or Final Tantra (*chima gyu*)

The four tantras are memorised in the order of the text, although the students' progress through the text does not match the sequence of lectures given in the Mentsikhang; students may be more advanced in the memorisation than in the topics covered by the lectures. This is considered to be the best learning method. Each semester, students are given deadlines for the memorisation of certain sections of the *Gyushi*, after which examinations are conducted in front of teachers and peers. During such examinations, students are asked to recite sections of the *Gyushi* for up to ten minutes.

In the first semester, students memorise the six chapters of the Root Tantra and its 'tree'. The tree is the arboreal 'map' of the tantra displayed on medical *thangkas* (Meyer, 1992). They also memorise chapters one to five and nine to eleven in the Explanatory Tantra, as well as the first half of 'The Golden Stalk: a condensed explanation of the culture of medicinal plants,'[6] a materia medica compendium by Kyenrab Norbu. They then memorise a grammar text and a Tibetan spelling treatise entitled 'Clarification of Spelling'.[7] In the second semester, students memorise much of the the Explanatory Tantra and its 'tree', chapters one to eleven of the Oral Instruction Tantra, and another grammar text.[8] During the third semester, students undertake the memorisation of chapters one to four and thirteen to thirty-one of the Oral Instruction Tantra, and of the anatomical treatise *byang khog yul thig* (literally meaning, 'lines of the chest'). They also study the writings from the Sakya sect of Tibetan Buddhism and the 'Letter to a Friend', a famous moral treatise composed by Nagarjuna.[9] In the fourth semester, students memorise several chapters and the 'tree' of the Final Tantra, as well as an outline of bloodletting points.[10] Finally, in the fifth semester, students learn the 'Lexicon of Medical Terms', the 'Explanation of Potencies' (a text about the effectiveness of different plants), and hymns in praise of Shakyamuni Buddha.[11]

As this brief description shows, Mentsikhang education focuses primarily on the *Gyushi*, its commentaries, and auxiliary texts. Some authors have argued that the heterogeneity of sources brought together in the *Gyushi* has created substantial tensions within the text, particularly between the theoretical content in the first tantras and the sections focusing on clinical practice contained in the last two tantras (Samuel, 2001). As was previously discussed, there has also been a tendency for doctors to leave out the more esoteric sections of the *Gyushi* and those dealing with traditional anatomy. The chapters are still taught in formal lectures and students are required to know their content. However, the deletion of specific chapters from the curriculum reflects a shift in medical practice.

Many sections from the *Gyushi*'s Explanatory Tantra are no longer memorised.[12] The majority of these deal with traditional Tibetan anatomy, physiology and medical instruments (including 'surgical' instruments). Similarly, the Mentsikhang teachers have discarded the majority of chapters dealing with classifications of the body and disorders. Interestingly, the two final chapters of the Explanatory Tantra, which explicitly deal with 'healing' (*so*) techniques and the role of the physician, have also been taken out of the curriculum.[13] These chapters specifically deal with the clinical aspects of medicine, for instance with the ways in which a doctor should make his or her speech soothing, and establish a relationship of trust with the patient to make sure he will continue treatment (*men che ten*).

The Oral Instruction Tantra is the least memorised of the four tantras: only a third of the ninety-two chapters are learnt by students today.[14] Two teachers and five students said that they still had to study the remaining chapters although memorising them was not needed. One female final-year student explained that this was because they had to know about 'old diseases' (*nying ne*). Her teachers did not share this view, and thought that accomplished practitioners should have a complete knowledge of the *Gyushi*. However, they admitted that the study of diseases like goitre was perhaps not so useful to contemporary students, and emphasised the value of experience or practice (*laglen*) in the making of a good practitioner.

The sections no longer memorised from the Quintessential Tantra were primarily descriptions of specific disorders and their causes, usually one or a combination of the three *nyepa*. In the curriculum, these disorders were unequivocally translated using biomedical terms. For instance, *drumpa* or pox was identified with smallpox, *yiga chupa* (repulsion with swallowing food) with anorexia, and *chinni* (Hindi for sugar) with diabetes. These diseases with specific biomedical aetiologies were left out of the Mentsikhang curriculum. The diseases that are still memorised are more complex general disorders relating to the digestive, pulmonary and hepatic systems (chapters thirty-four to fourty-one).

This gradual phasing out of the third tantra has been noted by Samuel, who argues that the tantra is 'at the core of how Tibetan doctors manage the transition between textual study and clinical practice, by clarifying many of the standard treatments and causes of commonly encountered diseases' (Samuel, 2001: 257–60). The fact that a large number of these diseases have been taken out of the compulsory curriculum may be read as a sign that Tibetan doctors in exile have grown cautious about labelling specific discrete illnesses, and feel more secure invoking general disorders of the Tibetan physiological system. Ambiguous disease categories that straddle biomedical and Tibetan aetiologies have been more or less replaced by biomedical ones, such as in the case of '*seje*', for which the biomedical category 'tuberculosis' is nowadays more frequently employed.

The Final Tantra's chapters on methods of diagnosis and treatment have also been subjected to a purge: only seven chapters out of twenty-seven are memorised today. These relate to pulse diagnosis, urine analysis, decoctions, powdered medicine, pills, and moxibustion.[15] Chapters from the *chima gyu* required for memorisation also correspond to the more common methods of diagnosis and treatment used by Mentsikhang doctors today. Other less popular treatments have been left out, as well as medicines less available in exile (like *rinpoche*, medicine with precious metals).

The Mentsikhang's recent publication of an additional textbook that reformulates principles explained in the Oral Instruction Tantra, the new 'Textbook of Tibetan Medicine', adjusts the *Gyushi*'s theoretical background to contemporary exile clinical practice.[16] Other texts, such as the 'Potencies of Medical Compounds',[17] are also reworking old categories in the light of new clinical needs and the growing influence of biomedicine. The 'Textbook', for example, brings in elements of biomedical anatomy and reworks some of the disease categories of the *Gyushi*'s third tantra.

Many of the transformations in Dharamsala's medical curriculum echo those made by Tibetan doctors in the Tibetan Autonomous Region (TAR). The TAR Mentsikhang has been prompt in incorporating new elements into medical training. For example, the medical dictionary 'The New Dawn Condensed Compendium of Healing Knowledge'[18] produced at Lhasa's Mentsikhang, presents modern anatomical drawings with both traditional and newly created Tibetan terms (*Samten*, 1997). It is available in India and commonly owned by younger Mentsikhang doctors. Gerke notes that 'compared to the traditional thangka paintings, [in contemporary Tibetan medical diagrams] there is a trend to be more detailed and accurate regarding gross anatomy … however, the subtle channels (*rtsa thig*) and invisible anatomy of the subtle body as depicted on the traditional thangkas do not appear here' (Gerke, 1998: 11). The aim of these new Tibetan medical textbooks is to impart a comparative knowledge of Tibetan and Western anatomy. The disappearance of the 'subtle channels' from the textbooks does not mean that doctors do not refer to them. In clinical practice, they still speak of disorders caused by damage or blocks in the *rtsa thig* ('subtle channels') that exist on the traditional Tibetan anatomical charts, although these do not appear in the new textbooks. The drawings in Figure 6.2 are examples of medical charts from the Tibet Autonomous Region that display Western anatomy with terminology adapted from the traditional Tibetan medical lexicon.

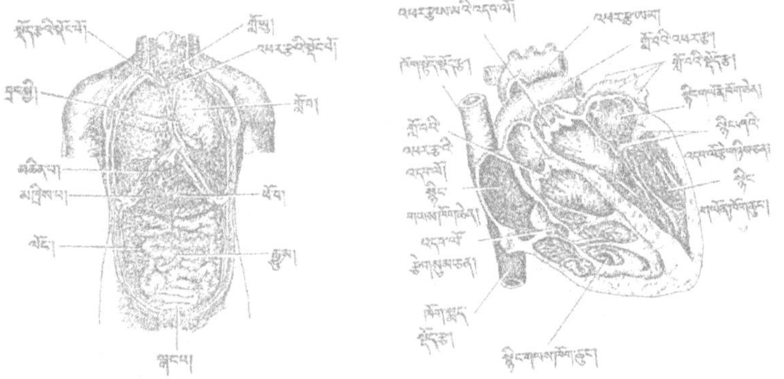

Figure 6.2: Anatomical drawings from *Gso rig snying bsdus skya phrengs gsar pa* (The New Dawn Condensed Compendium of Healing Knowledge), manual published by the Lhasa Mentsikhang in 1997.

In the first drawing, depicting the anatomy of a human chest (*dankog*), the terms identifying traditional organ systems have been retained, although they now designate discrete organs rather than systems or channels, as in older anatomical depictions.[19]

The second anatomical drawing depicts a human heart and presents some interesting medical terminology: the aorta is refered to as the *partsa ama* ('mother great' external vein), and *partsa* is used in equivalence to the term 'artery' (as it is in contemporary translations of older medical texts (Meyer, 1992). The word for petal (*dablo*) is used to refer to 'valves'. Much of this new terminology recycles the vocabulary of more traditional Tibetan anatomy and its arboreal metaphors (with roots, trunks, stems and petals). There is, however, a clear contrast between contemporary Lhasa Mentsikhang charts, which make use of biomedical anatomy with Tibetan medical neologisms, and former Tibetan anatomy charts, such as the thangkas displayed in Meyer (1992).

In parallel to this disappearance of traditional Tibetan anatomy, some concepts present in older medical texts have been given new salience because of their resemblance to biomedical notions. For instance, *sin*, which was previously used to refer to parasites or demons, is now commonly translated in Tibetan medical books as 'microorganism'. It regularly finds its way into discussion of infectious diseases as a term designating biological disease agents (as does the word *bu sin*, referring to insects or worms, which is now often used to designate the concept of 'germ').

In parallel to this 'recycling' of older Tibetan medical terms, new words have been coined to describe organs that did not previously exist in traditional Tibetan anatomy. Gerke (1998: 11) notes that the Tibetan word for pancreas (*sherma*) was only created in the twentieth century. With the rising prevalence of diabetes in Tibetan settlements, increased emphasis was given to a biomedical model that ascribes the cause of diabetes to a dysfunction of the pancreas, as opposed to a model rooted in the imbalance of the three humours.

The selective use of curricular texts, the creation of 'hybrid' textbooks combining traditional Tibetan medical theory with biomedical anatomy, and the renewal of the traditional anatomical language to fit changes in clinical practice are reflections of ongoing changes in

Tibetan medicine. I would suggest that these changes partly stem from the radically different circumstances of clinical practice in exile. Present exile circumstances are making links between the environment and disease more tangible. Tibetan medicine is now in a liminal phase: current disease categories and treatment methods are being reworked, while older ones are being eroded and even voluntarily discarded. An example of this 're-creation' of disease categories will be examined in detail in the final section of this chapter with the treatment of diabetes.

Tibetan medical knowledge transmission outside the Mentsikhang

Although Tibetan medicine is practised today in Bhutan, Mongolia, Tibet, and the Indian states of Himachal Pradesh, Ladakh and Sikkim, its 'styles' differ between institutions and individuals. Historically, the transmission of medical knowledge through lineages is the oldest form of learning and teaching in Tibetan medicine. In Ladakh, it is customary for medical knowledge to be transmitted from father to son, or mother to daughter. However, with recent local developments in medical training, Ladakhi traditional healers, or *amchis*, have broken away from this tradition and started recruiting apprentices among young locals. Such programmes are meant to create a broader recruitment base for *amchi* training and aim to make their knowledge relevant to the provision of primary health-care in the more remote provinces of the region, such as Zanskar. In recent years however, Mentsikhang doctors have begun to brand hereditary knowledge transmission as 'unprofessional'. Many believe that hereditarily trained practitioners do not have to work hard to inherit a title from their parents, and feel that institutional training is a safer way of ensuring the quality of medical education.

Another factor that seems to have influenced this growing difference in 'styles' between the Mentsikhang and independent doctors is the emergence of Tibetan medical clinics that cater principally to foreigners. The great majority of foreigners who try Tibetan medicine in Dharamsala have no knowledge of its diagnostic techniques and theoretical underpinnings. Having one urine's analysed is often considered the 'high point' of a consultation, the climactic moment of this 'exotic' medical encounter (Rabgay, 1994b). Whereas Mentsikhang doctors seldom practice urine analysis for routine consultations, in a private Tibetan clinic such as Dr Yeshi Donden's, patients are told that they have to come with an empty stomach and having drunk some water, so that they can provide the required urine at their morning consultation. Ironically, for some foreign patients, this hallmark of Tibetan medicine becomes reminiscent of experiences in Western clinics, where they have to come in on an empty stomach before surgery.

Tibetan medicine, when practised 'on' foreigners, works paradoxically. On the one hand, it seeks to enforce an impression of authenticity by privileging a mode of diagnosis regarded as 'traditional' and uniquely Tibetan. On the other, through its clinical practice, it invites comparisons with the procedural rigidity of biomedicine.

The famed physician Yeshi Donden receives more than fifty patients every morning in his private McLeod clinic.[20] According to his foreign patients, he carries out urine analysis on a virtually automatic basis, in an almost 'ultra-traditional' style of practice. During my own consultation, Dr Donden poured the urine into a white 'examination bowl', inspected it thoroughly by looking for bubbles and scrutinising its colouring. To the foreign patient, he almost seems to 'divine' the patient's health status from the bowl's contents. One India-born Tibetan recalled a particularly itchy problem, which he went to report to Dr Yeshi Donden in his McLeod Ganj practice:

> This was at a time when there were announcements on the Indian radio, I think it was after some numbers about rape were published and the government was becoming worried about the increase of violence against women in the country. There were these series of announcements by a doctor, a sex specialist, saying that for men to do it themselves [i.e, masturbate] was a good thing, it relieved tension and so they didn't turn against women. It was healthy. I thought this was probably true so I started doing it. Then a few months later, I started to get this itchy sensation ... down there. So I went to see Dr Yeshi Donden, because I thought there was something really wrong with me. So when I came to the clinic, he asked me to pull down my trousers. I was really embarrassed, but I had to do it. Then he looked at me for

about three minutes, looking at everything! He didn't say anything but asked to see the sample of urine I had brought with me. After tasting the urine, he simply asked if I had been, you know, doing a lot recently. I laughed and said yes. He didn't give me any medicine but just told me to stop doing so much for a while. You can't fool Dr. Yeshi Donden, he knows what is wrong with you.*

The fast pace at which a famed doctor like Yeshi Donden sees patients usually doesn't allow for a great deal of elaboration on each case. However, some doctors will regularly see the same patients and frequent patients to the Mentsikhang have their personal doctors.

In addition to these encounters with foreign patients in Dharamsala, numerous Tibetan doctors, both Dharamsala and TAR-trained, have found asylum in the West, where they practise in institutions or privately. There are Tibetan practitioners in Italy, Switzerland, Germany, the UK (including the Tara College of Tibetan Medicine in Samye Ling, Scotland), Sweden, Denmark, and the USA. Tibetan doctors practising abroad have had great difficulties in cultivating or importing medical substances, sometimes even leading to legal problems when they have tried to obtain medical substances for their patients. Tibetan medical doctors from the Mentsikhang and other Tibetan institutions in India also regularly come to Europe and America to lecture on Tibetan medicine.

Some exiled doctors have well-established clinics, which have developed a 'style' of Tibetan medical practice tailored to Western patients. Dr Dickey, a TAR-born female doctor, advertises her practice in Berkeley, California, in the following way:[21]

Dr Dickey is a *seventh* generation Tibetan physician (her uncle was a physician to His Holiness the Dalai Lama). Her family's mission is to preserve and promote the ancient and mystical yet highly effective holistic ways of Tibet's healing heritage as she gives workshops and consultations seeing clients around the States as well as the clinic in Berkeley. She hopes to establish a Tibetan Medical school in the West.

ABOUT DR DICKEY:

Dr Dickey, TMD is a traditional doctor of Tibetan Medicine. She is the sole practising female Tibetan physician in the United States today. Her family name is synonymous with compassionate medical care in her homeland Tibet. While her early training in medicine was in the

Nyerongsha Medical School (as a young girl at age seven she began studying pulses etc.), she graduated from Mentsikhang, the most prestigious medical school in Lhasa, Tibet. Dr Dickey maintains consulting practices in Colorado, Arizona, Texas, and throughout California as well. She resides in San Francisco.

The description lists what is required of the patient coming for a consultation:

1) NO medications except for necessary prescriptions
2) NO red meat
3) NO alcohol
4) NO coffee
5) NO black tea
6) NO vitamins
7) NO foods that are unusual to your normal diet
8) NO nutritional yeast
9) NO strenuous activity
10) NO sexual activity
11) NO beets, asparagus or red Swiss chard
12) NO shower or bath in the morning before your appointment

Dr Dickey has clearly appropriated a biomedical doctor's garb, while trying to accentuate the traditional and holistic allure of her practice: she has given herself a hybrid but institutional sounding title, 'TMD', which may ambiguously stand for 'Traditional' or 'Tibetan' Medical Doctor. She lists an extensive number of prerequisites for the consultation, thereby communicating an impression of clinical efficacy. Dr Dickey refers to an established familial medical tradition, institutional legitimacy (the Lhasa Mentsikhang degree), and an affiliation with the Dalai Lama. She appears to be keen to draw a connection between her own 'style' of medical practice and the aspects of Tibetan culture that the West is most familiar with, namely Buddhism and the Dalai Lama. By doing so, she deliberately accentuates the association of Tibetan medicine with spirituality and holism. She is also further legitimating her own status as a 'traditional' practitioner in a setting where alternative medicines abound and compete with each other to earn the cachet of 'authenticity'.

One biomedical term, many Tibetan symptoms

Although learning specific biomedical terms is not actively encouraged by the Mentsikhang, students and doctors who interact with Western patients often make their own tables of biomedical/Tibetan equivalences through books and through their own clinical experience. This is allegedly so that they may be able to explain their prognosis to foreign patients, but, in my experience, it is also simply a result of professional curiosity.

But direct translation and equivalence-making between Tibetan medical syndromes and biomedical diseases is hazardous: Tibetan medicine sometimes defines a disease by its causes or symptoms without giving it the name of an actual condition, while sometimes regrouping a set of diverse symptoms under one term. An example of this is the gynaecological disease *lung tshabs*, which refers to an excess of *lung* humour in the womb, but can cover a vast array of problems ranging from infertility to hysteria. This problem is accentuated by contemporary doctors' use of Western terms to gloss over Tibetan disorders. One Tibetan doctor from Mentsikhang commonly used the term 'spondylitis' to describe damage inflicted to his *tsa karpo* (which he translated as sciatic nerve) by sitting uncomfortably under a cool fan for long hours. The students' rapid adoption of biomedical terminology is an indicator of the Mentsikhang's increasing contact with biomedical doctors and foreign patients. This is also manifested in the Mentsikhang's adoption of Latin botanical terms for the majority of prescribed medicine and medical products.

Doctors have different views on the systematised translation of Tibetan disorder names into biomedical terms. One male doctor who had been involved in a 'clinical trial' project on diabetes said that he found the use of biomedical terms 'safer' when dealing with biomedical doctors. His fear was that they would not understand references to the three humours, and might be misled by literal translations of traditional Tibetan anatomy. Another male student, perhaps more 'traditionally' inclined, told me that that the new system of transliterating biomedical terms phonetically in the Tibetan alphabet (for example *diyabitis* for diabetes) would be more appropriate. He explained that Dharamsala doctors should not change their practice simply because clinical tests were being performed. He did not believe the tests would 'prove' anything, largely because they were looking for disorders in different 'systems' (*lug*). This student also reflected on the poor practice of some doctors who had become used to prescribing pills without trying to pinpoint the exact causes of disease through interrogation, but simply by recognising typical sets of symptoms. This, he claimed, was a result of poor motivation.

Tibetan doctors are now stressing the importance of differentiating between Tibetan disorders and biomedical diseases with similar symptoms and aetiologies. For instance, practitioners insist on differentiating the Tibetan disorder *chinni ne* (lit. sugar disease) from diabetes, now commonly referred to as *diyabitis*. However, monks I spoke to about their diabetes treatment at Delek Hospital invariably referred to the condition as *chinni natsa*, which shows that, although the distinction may hold among medical practitioners, it is still not uniformly adopted by the 'lay' community.

Doctors and students see the translation of Tibetan medical terms into biomedical ones as largely hazardous. Reasons for this are two-fold. Doctors involved in the Mentsikhang's research activities and clinical trials have been confronted with the legal and epistemological difficulties arising from hastily drawn equivalences. Problems specifically arise when high expectations about the efficacy of Tibetan medicine are combined with the ascription of biomedical categories to diseases treated by Tibetan doctors (as in the case of hepatitis B). Tibetan doctors are now emphasising the differences between traditional Tibetan and biomedical physiology. The growing popularity of Tibetan medicine has heightened the general level of knowledge of its aetiological premises, and Mentsikhang doctors are gaining confidence in using their own terminology rather than biomedical terms.

In recent years, the Mentsikhang has begun to research the clinical efficacy of its compounds against conditions such as hepatitis B and diabetes. However, the design of clinical trials for Tibetan medicine poses a number of epistemological, ethical and practical problems. Epistemologically, the difficulty lies in determining suitable outcomes for clinical trials, since Tibetan medicine operates holistically and does not treat diseases 'in isolation'. Furthermore, the timing of outcome measurements is also problematic: Tibetan medicine is thought to act more slowly on the body than biomedicine. There have also been ethical queries concerning the relevance of clinical trials in the assessment of traditional medical systems.[22] Social scientists, in particular, have criticised the use of randomised clinical trials (RCTs) to evaluate traditional compounds. Some have argued that RCTs unfairly shift the ownership of medical knowledge out of practitioners' hands and into those of the corporations and states financing trials. Adams (2002c), for example, has shown that the financial interest generated by 'exotic' Tibetan medicines in China has led to randomised controlled trials designed to prove the efficacy of discrete, marketable 'active ingredients', thereby contradicting the holistic outlook of Tibetan medicine and robbing Tibetan physicians of their intellectual property.

As the market for Tibetan medicine continues to expand in China, a paradox emerges: political and financial pressures are exerted on doctors to prove scientific efficacy while, at the same time, consumers are encouraged to believe in the 'exotic' and 'magical' properties of Tibetan medicines. It is in the context of this Chinese backdrop that exile doctors negotiate the design of clinical trials for their own compounds.

Researching traditional medicine and proving authenticity

A few years before my fieldwork, a trial had been conducted to explore the efficacy of Tibetan medicine as an adjunct to treatment for diabetes mellitus (Namdul et al., 2001). In this trial, physicians faced pragmatic difficulties in terms of study design. What should be the criteria used to measure efficacy? Should the measured outcomes only take into account the curative properties of plants or should they also encompass the holistic approach characteristic of Tibetan medicine, which includes an evaluation of diet and lifestyle? There were also a number of practical and epistemological issues, for example, the difficulty of truly randomising patients in the context of small communities, and of devising placebos when traditional doctors did not consider any medical compound to be inactive.

In a colloquium held at the Mentsikhang in 1996, a multicultural team prepared a protocol for the clinical trial. The team of traditional Tibetan doctors refused the single drug tests and modified the project's guidelines to incorporate diet and behavioural regimen with multi-drug use.[23] In other words, the possibility of a more conventional clinical drug trial was effectively ruled out because the holistic approach used in Tibetan medicine would not allow a single therapeutic protocol for diabetes mellitus. The term 'clinical trial' was retained, however, because the outcomes measured were not the Tibetan medical criteria, but rather blood-glucose levels.

According to the *Gyushi*, there are several causes and types of *diyabitis*. The basic causal factors are excessive production of fats and phlegm (*beygen*) in the body due to over-consumption of foods dominated by the earth (*sa*) and water (*chu*) elements. According to the physician Pema Dorjee, 'The substance formed by such predominance of elements is cold (*tangmo*) in potency and sweet (*ngarmo*) in taste (*ro*). Due to its antagonistic potency, the heat (*dö*) of the digestive fire gets degenerated and results in weakness of digestion' (Dorjee, 1984: 4). Thus, the main aim of treatment is to restore digestive functions so that food will be well assimilated by the body.

Mentsikhang doctors designed the trial protocol in collaboration with a Delhi-based research laboratory. It was referred to as a double blind randomised controlled clinical trial of diabetes mellitus, and its stated objective was 'to assess the efficacy of Tibetan medicine in controlling the plasma glucose and glycated hemoglobin (GHb) in newly diagnosed or untreated type 2 diabetes mellitus'. The study lasted from April 1997 to March 2000. In 1997, a group of doctors from the Mentsikhang took the significant decision to extend the trial from a 'single drug study' to a 'multiple drug study', which would be more suitable considering to the Tibetan method of prescribing more than one kind of pill or compound for a given condition. The study's outcomes included changes in patients' self-perceived well-being, relief from symptoms (defined as a decrease in blood glucose), change in weight or blood pressure, and the appearance of new complaints. There was no mention of assessing the patient's humoral imbalance as reflected in the pulse. The researchers used strictly biomedical measurements.[23]

In the trial, 200 newly diagnosed diabetes patients were randomly allocated to the intervention or to a control group. The intervention group took Tibetan medicine in the form of powder or pills with dietary and lifestyle modification advice adapted from the American Diabetes Association. The second group followed the same dietary and lifestyle modification advice but did not receive any medication. Patients were given a physical examination twelve and twenty-four weeks into the trial.

The pills used in the treatment of patients were Kyuru 6, Yungwa 4, Chenyi Aru 18, and Sugmel 19. Kyuru 6 was prescribed to all patients, along with at least two of the other medicines. The choice of treatment regimen depended on the severity of the case. Severity was determined using traditional Tibetan diagnosis techniques (urine or pulse diagnosis) and by measuring blood-glucose levels at baseline. Doctors also made modifications to the treatment if they found notable changes in blood-glucose levels twelve weeks into the trial. The herbal pill regimen was not subject to individual tailoring and the Tibetan doctors attempted to standardise treatment as much as possible.

It is clear from the methodology devised that the experiment sought to verify the biological properties of 'active ingredients' within Tibetan medicine. Little concern had in fact been given to the other essential aspects of treatment in Tibetan medicine, such as the individual tailoring of treatment in accordance to diet and lifestyle. Moreover, the potential placebo effects of traditional medicine were not taken into account.

Eighty-two out of the 200 patients recruited to the study withdrew invoking 'social reasons'. Only two patients complained that their symptoms had worsened after treatment. Overall, the trial was declared a success: biomedical observers noted a decrease in fasting and postprandial plasma glucose in the group treated with Tibetan medicine.[24] The researchers concluded that taking Tibetan medicine along with exercise and diet was more effective in controlling glycaemic levels than exercise and diet alone.

However, Tibetan doctors had been forced into a number of compromises in order to comply with the requirements of this clinical trial. They reduced the benefits of their medical practice to the efficacy of herbal substances. The trial protocol also limited their clinical freedom in order to standardise treatment procedures. Many of the alleged benefits of Tibetan medicine therefore became lost in the trade-off for a biomedically sound trial.

In exile as in the TAR, the use of RCTs has the effect of transferring the 'ownership' of knowledge away from doctors and into the hands of institutions and companies that fund and design trials. The commercialisation of Tibetan medicine hinges on a double proof: first, that of clinical efficacy, with the subsequent race for trials and search for 'active ingredients'; and secondly, that of 'authenticity', which is achieved through the use of elaborate packaging and marketing techniques evoking the 'magic' of Tibetan medicine (Adams, 2002c).

However, the Dharamsala Mentsikhang has more freedom to retain traditional practices than its TAR counterpart, partly because its stated aim is the preservation of 'Tibetan traditional knowledge'. Although it is also under pressure to demonstrate clinical efficacy, the Mentsikhang gains considerable credibility from the Dalai Lama's endorsement. Furthermore, the religious underpinnings of Tibetan medicine are relatively unproblematic in exile, unlike in the TAR. This aids Tibetan physicians who wish to demonstrate the connection between their medical and their religious practices.

By addressing key exile problems such as the emergence of *lung* or disorders linked to the environmental changes, the Mentsikhang also plays a key role in fostering 'public health' in the Tibetan community. Its physicians seek to redress the imbalances generated by the move to exile. Patients also think of the Mentsikhang as a guardian of Tibetan knowledge and Buddhist values, which makes its physicians able to diagnose and treat Tibetan-specific disorders such as *lung*. The Mentsikhang's role in strengthening public health is also readily evidenced in the production and distribution of *rilbu* at public gatherings. *Rilbu* made at the Mentsikhang and blessed by lamas are given out to Tibetans with the clear aim of strengthening their health and conferring Buddhist blessings. The Mentsikhang is therefore, at a community level, an essential player in health promotion.

Notes

1. Tibetan medicine was officially sanctioned as a component of the health system in India in 1962. The Mentsikhang now has the status of 'charitable association' under the patronage of the Dalai Lama and does not pay income tax to the Indian government, though it does pay taxes on export sales. At the time of fieldwork (2000–2002), there were three other relatively large institutions teaching Tibetan medicine in India. The first was the 'Institute of Tibetan Medicine' run by Dr Tashigang in New Delhi. The second, Chagpori Institute in Darjeeling, was founded in 1992 by one of few remaining lineage holders of the Chagpori College, Trogawa Rinpoche. Although the Chagpori Institute retains a certain amount of independence with regard to teachings, its curriculum roughly mirrors that of the Mentsikhang and Chagpori students have to take their final exams at the Mentsikhang if they are to be awarded the degree of *sman pa ka chu pa*. The third training institution for Tibetan medicine was the medical department established as part of the Central Institute for Higher Tibetan Studies in Sarnath in 1993. All three institutions now follow the same curriculum of five years of study in the school and two years of clinical training, corresponding roughly to that of the Mentsikhang.
2. The term *nyams rtogs* is also used in a religious context to designate meditation experiences in Buddhism.
3. Millard, in a study of 'learning processes' in a West Nepal Tibetan Bonpo medical school (2002), outlines the progression that leads students from relying on propositional memory (with an emphasis on memorisation), to an increasing use of procedural memory (with an emphasis on skills).
4. The medicine Buddha resides at the centre of the mandala on a throne made of lapis lazuli. He is dark blue, a colour that reflects the diseases he has taken upon him and is able to cure. He holds a begging bowl in his left hand and a *myrobalan* (great medicine plant) in his right hand.
5. The yearly trip to nearby mountains and Manali is seen by Mentsikhang students as one of the highlights of the year.
6. '*Sngo sman 'khrung dpe sdus pa ngo mtshar gser gyi snyi ma*'.
7. '*Dka' gnad gsal sgron*' and '*Dag yig ngag sgron*'.
8. '*Si tu'i drel chen*'.
9. '*Sa kya legs bshad*' and '*bShes pa'i spring yig*'.
10. '*Gzhon nu'i ngag rgyan*'.
11. '*Sman ming brda sprod*', '*Sman sbyor nus pa phyogs bsdus phan bde'i legs bshad*' by Tobtsen Jedrub, and '*Khyad par 'phags stod*'.
12. These include *dra dpe* (3: similes of the body); *lus kyi gnas lugs* (4: anatomy); *lus kyi las dang dbye ba* (6: actions and classifications of the body); *cha byad dpyad* (21: medical instruments); *mi na gnas ston* (22: normal health); *nyes pa dngos ston* (23: techniques for correct diagnosis);

ngan gyo skyon brtag (24: techniques for gaining a patient's confidence); *spang blang mu bzhi* (25: four diagnostic techniques to verify if the patient can be healed or not); *gso thabs gnos* (29: the healing techniques); *sman pa'i le'u* (30: chapter on the healer physician).

13. In reality, *so* (Wylie spelling: *gsos*) is a complex term: etymologically, it encompasses activities as diverse as feeding, nourishing, rearing, mending, repairing and curing. As the verbalised clause *gso bar byed*, it relates more specifically to medical treatment, with references to curing or putting an end to disease (Das, 1902: 1312).
14. Chapters memorised include: *zhus pa* (1: request for the teaching of the Oral Instruction Tantra); *rlung* (2: diagnosis and treatment of rlung disorders); *mkhris pa* (3: diagnosis and treatment of *mkhris pa* disorders); *bad kan* (4: diagnosis and treatment of bad kan disorders); *tsha grang gal mdo* (13: method to distinguish between hot and cold disorders); *tsha ba ri thang mtshams* (14: method to distinguish the border, or *tshams*, between hot and cold disorder); chapters 34–41 comprising *snying nad, glo nad, mchin nad, mcher nad, mkhal nad, pho ba'i nad, rgyu ma'i nad* and *long nad* (namely disorders of the heart, lungs, liver, spleen, kidneys, stomach, small intestine and large intestine). The final chapters of the Oral Instruction Tantra, which deal mostly with 'psychiatric' disorders are memorised in the fifth semester of teaching (78: *smyo byed*, insanity; *brjed byed*, amnesia; *gza'*, epilepsy, etc.).
15. *rtsa* (pulse diagnosis); *chu* (urine diagnosis); *thang* (decoction); *phye ma* (powdered medicine); *ril bu* (pills); *gtar* (blood letting); *bsreg* (moxibustion).
16. '*Gso rig lob dpe*'.
17. '*Sman jor gyi nus pa*'.
18. '*Gso ba rig pa'i tsig mdzod gyu thog dgongs rgyan*'.
19. There are references to the *glo ba* (lung), *mchin pa* (liver), *mkhris pa* (in this case the gall bladder), *pho ba* (stomach), *long* (gut), *rgyu ma* (instestine), and *lgang pa* (urinary bladder). *dab lo rtse gsum can* (literally, the point endowed with three petals), designates the tricuspid valve.
20. Dr Donden was the first director of the MTK (1961–66) before going into private practice.
21. See www.siamsewana.org/phpBB2/viewtopic.php?t=484 (accessed 26 July 2007).
22. In the UK, the General Medical Council gives traditional medicines legal status on the basis of ascertainable, long-standing practice, while encouraging research through clinical trials to ensure the safety of products prescribed. See also, the WHO's 'General Guidelines for Methodologies on Research and Evaluation of Traditional Medicine', http://whqlibdoc.who.int/hq/2000/WHO_EDM_TRM_2000.1.pdf. (accessed 26 July 2007).

23. The Mentsikhang has also reportedly been engaged in herbal research for treatments against cancer, and has set up a three-month camp in Dharamsala with the Cancer Detection Society of India to 'incorporate the indigenous Tibetan medical system into the detection and cure of cancer as part of a holistic multidisciplinary approach'. The MTK has also held 'Breast Cancer Camps' with the help of visiting Indian doctors, responding to the increasing fear of breast cancer in the community.
24. According to Dr Namdul, (Namdul et al., 2001), the trial endpoints were: 1. Fasting Plasma Glucose (PG) less than 140 mg/dl; 2. postprandial PG less than 200 mg/dl; 3.glycated haemoglobin (GHb) less than 8.5%.

Epilogue

This book has sought to address two salient issues: first, the impact of social inequalities on health in the Tibetan settlements; and, secondly, Tibetan traditional medicine's role in maintaining public health in exile communities.

Drawing on thirteen months of ethnographic fieldwork among Tibetans in India, I have shown how the Mentsikhang, the Tibetans' primary traditional medical institution in exile, has adapted its practice to the needs of the exile population. Tibetan physicians have become particularly apt at diagnosing disorders associated with exile (for example increases in *lung*), and disorders linked to changes in climate and diet. Moreover, Mentsikhang physicians have changed the teaching curriculum to place emphasis on clinical methods relevant to contemporary practice. They have also discarded or modified disease categories when these invited direct competition with biomedicine, for example, 'diabetes' or 'hepatitis B'. While attempting to negotiate their status in relation to biomedicine, for instance, by complying with trial methodologies, Tibetan physicians attempt to retain their autonomy by defending traditional clinical categories. The Mentsikhang also plays a considerable role in supporting the political will to preserve health: by distributing *mani rilbu* in political gatherings and engaging in the care of newcomers and torture survivors, Mentsikhang physicians make a critical contribution to exile public health.

For individual exiles, illness is often understood in terms of place-based disorder or contagion. This concern is echoed in traditional Tibetan medical practice, which places particular emphasis on the seasonal, dietary and behavioural determinants of illness. The economic and political context of exile has also impacted on the way in which traditional Tibetan medicine is taught and practised: a more systematised and institutionalised system has been put in place by the

Mentsikhang to defend its status as the main provider of Tibetan medicine in exile. The political role given to the Mentsikhang by the Tibetan government in exile further entrenches this status. The official stamp of approval also contributes to Tibetan traditional medicine's 'symbolic efficacy' by making it a communal resource, and, as Janes described in the context of the TAR, 'a fund for ethnic revitalisation'. At a symbolic level, the 'unhealthy' state of exile has led to an increase in the Tibetan community's moral investment in Tibetan medicine. Tibetan medicine is also politically validated as authentically Tibetan and, as such, participates in the project of cultural survival that is so vital to the public health of exiles.

Tibetan medicine 'works' in exile, I argue, not only because its practice is predicated upon a careful consideration of changes in local environmental factors, but also because it goes on to shape people's understandings of health in practice. Where the local social landscape is deeply affected by political struggle, such as in the Tibetan situation, traditional medicines become a resource for public health through their work as 'emplacing' practices. By 'adjusting' Tibetan exile bodies to the environment of exile, Tibetan medicine emplaces a displaced community.

The second point made in this book relates to the importance of examining social inequalities within diaspora communities. When we think of health inequalities and diasporas, we tend to think of inequalities between diaspora communities and host groups. Typically, unrelenting discrimination and social inequalities between diaspora and host communities result in persistent health inequities. However, little consideration has been given to the consequences of socio-economic inequalities within diasporas on health. Within diaspora communities, some social groups may be more affected by socio-economic deprivation, lack of access to health-care and stigma than others. Moreover, diasporic 'imaginations', or culturally shaped discourses about diaspora and the homeland, are fashioned by, and contribute to, ideas about health and health inequalities. Migration may contribute to the erosion of social solidarity and to poor mental health as well as facilitate the spread of infectious diseases, in what has been called a 'pathogenic social spiral' (Nguyen and Peschard, 2003). This book has sought to demonstrate that such a phenomenon is appearing within the Tibetan exile community. The growing socio-economic rift between 'old-timers' and newcomers is causing health inequalities, with more newcomers diagnosed with communicable diseases such as tuberculosis, and suffering from Tibetan disorders linked to anxiety and mental strain, such as *lung*. As anthropologists return time and time again to the consequences, both local and global, of social inequalities (Farmer 1997, 2003), attention needs to be paid to inequalities within diaspora communities, and to the ways in which internal and external inequalities interact to influence health.

Looking north to the Tibet Autonomous Region and Tibetan cultural areas, Tibetan medicine is poised for radical changes (Adams et al., 2005). In the TAR, investments in Tibetan medicine are directly linked to socialist ambitions for a sinicised Tibet; Buddhism and the Tibetan cultural heritage, of which medicine is an integral part, are tolerated as long as they can be marketed. In India, on the other hand, Tibetan medicine is endorsed as a powerful resource to promote public health among refugees: it has become a vehicle for messages about physical and moral health at a time of political uncertainty. Traditional medicine remains at the heart of the struggle to define modern Tibetan identities.

Glossary of Tibetan Words with Wylie Spellings

This glossary uses the Wylie (1959) transliteration system without hyphenation. All words in italics are in the Wylie spelling. Capitalisation of the first letter is used for names (e.g., *Sde srid sangs rgyas rgya mthso*), titles (e.g., *Zhi khro dgongs pa rang grol*), and places (e.g. *Bsam yas*). In some instances the capitalised letter will be an unpronounced prefix letter (e.g., in *Glang dar ma*) and the phonetic rendition should be used for pronounciation (Langdarma).

Bardo thodol (*Bar do thos grol*)
Literally, 'Liberation upon hearing in the Bardo.' This text is best known as 'The Tibetan Book of the Dead', from the '*Zhi khro dgongs pa rang grol*', or 'The self-liberated mind of the peaceful and wrathful ones', a text revealed by Karma Lingpa.

Beygen (*bad kan*)
Phlegm humour, one of the bodily aspects or humours

Beygen mugpo (*bad kan smug po*)
'Brown' phlegm

Bhaisajyaguru (*sman bla*)
Medicine Buddha

Bö shung mentsikhang (*bod gzhung sman rtsis khang*)
Tibetan Government Astro-Medical Institute

Bu (*'bu*)
Microorganism, parasite, bacteria

Bu sin (*'bu srin*)
Insect, parasite

Chagpori (*Lcags po ri*)
Literally 'Iron mountain', the name of the hill on which the traditional Tibetan medical college in Lhasa was situated. Tibetans call it *Sman rtsi khang* or *Bod sman slob grwa chen mo*. A new medical college by the name of Chagpori Medical Institute was founded in Darjeeling (India) in 1992.

Cha karpo tungwa (*ja gar po 'thung ba*)
To drink strong tea

Champa (*cham pa*)
Cold, influenza

Chang, arak (*chang, a rag*)
Alcohol (local barley beer and Indian alcohol)

Changlug (*byang lugs*)
Northern school of Tibetan medicine

Chima gyu (*Phyi ma'i rgyud*)
The final tantra of the *Gyushi*

Ching (*bying*)
Sunken (pulse)

Chin ne (*mchin nad*)
Liver disease

Chinpa (*mchin pa*)
Liver

Chu (*chu*)
Water

Churwa (*chur ba*)
Cheese

Cu med se che (*bcud med zas spyad*)
Under-eating

Dablo (*'dab lo*)
Valves, petals, leaves

Dag shin (*bdag 'dzin*)
Self-grasping, ego

Damaru (*da ma ru*)
Small hand drum

Damtsig (*dam tshig*)
Binding vow

Dangkog (*brang khog*)
Human chest

Da tsen (*zla mtshan*)
Period

Dö (*drod*)
Heat

Dochag (*'dod chags*)
Attachment, lust, passion

Dogong (*dud khung*)
A chimney

Dokhog shelwa (*grod khog bshal ba*)
Diarrhoea

Don (*gdon*)
Malevolent spirit

Drilbu (*dril bu*)
Bell

Drip (*grib*)
Contamination

Drumpa (*'brum pa*)
Grain, small particle, pox, or smallpox (*'brum nad* or *lha 'brum* are also used for smallpox)

Dung gyu (*gdung rgyud*)
Lineage

Dze ne (*mdze nad*)
Leprosy

Gangchen Kyishong (*Gangs can skyid gshongs*)
Middle settlement of Dharamsala, where the Mentsikhang and Delek Hospital are located

Geka (*rgas ka*)
Old age

Go ne (*mgo nad*)
Headaches

Gowa'i bu (*'go ba'i 'bu*)
Infectious *bu*

Gul cham (*mgul cham*)
A cold (sore) throat

Gyagka (*gyag kha*)
Foul mouth (slang)

Gyalwa rinpoche (*rgyal ba rin po che*)
The 'precious victorious one', a common epithet for His Holiness the Dalai Lama

Gyupa (*rgyud pa*)
Lineage (e.g. lineage of teachers of Tibetan medicine)

Gyushi (*Rgyud bzhi*)
Four Medical Tantras

Injiy (*dbyin ji*)
A commonly used term for foreigners

Jinden (*byin rten*)
Protective substances, relics

Kala (*kha lag*)
Food. See also: *kha lag ma gtsang*, unclean food; *kha lag snum pa*, oily/fatty food; *kha lag rul ba*, rotten food; *kha lag grang mo*, cold food; *kha lag thal za ba*, overeating; *kha lag tsha po, skyur po za ba*, eating hot and sour food; *kha lag mngar mo*, sweet food

Kam marpo (*khams dmar po*)
Red element (in human reproduction)

Katam (*kha gtam*)
Lectures, oral tradition

Katon don (*kha ton 'don*)
Recitation

Katon du she pa (*kha ton du shes pa*)
To know by heart, to be able to recite; an important skill in medical and monastic learning

Kel ne (*mkhal nad*)
Kidney disorder

Kepo (*mkhas po*)
Expert

Khorlo (*'khor lo*)
Key points in the subtle anatomy of the body (Sanskrit: chakra)

Kimtsang (*khyim tsang*)
Extended family

Korlam (*skor lam*)
Circumambulation path

Ku (*sku*)
The physical body

Kuche (*sku mched*)
Brothers and sisters

Ku kam (*sku khams*)
A healthy bodily state

Ku kar (*sku mkhar*)
A royal fortress

Ku ring (*sku ring*)
Lifetime. The terms lifespan (*tshe ring po*) and longevity (*sku tshe*) are also used.

Kushog (*sku gzhogs*)
Honorific for 'person'; also often used in reference to monks.

Kushog dengdu (*sku gzhogs deng dus*)
Modern monk

Kuwa (*khu ba*)
Reproductive substances

Kyab solwa (*skyabs bcol ba*)
Refugee, someone who seeks refuge from harm

Kyangma (*rkyang ma*)
The left channel

Kyen (*rkyen*)
Secondary causes, as opposed to rgyu or primary cause

Kyo ngelwa (*skyo ngal ba*)
Sadness

Laglen (*lag len*)
Practice

Lama (*bla ma*)
Teacher

Le (*las*)
Karma, the law of cause and effect in Tibetan Buddhism

Le ki lung (*las kyi rlung*)
The wind of karma

Le ngen (*las ngan*)
Negative karma

Lo'i natsa (*glo'i na tsha*)
Lung disorder

Losar (*lo gsar*)
Tibetan New Year

Lug (*lugs*)
Approach, system, method, tradition

Lugar (*glu gar*)
Song and dance performances

Luki nupa (*lus kyi nus pa*)
Bodily strength

Lu malong (*lus ma long pa*)
Bodily discomforts

Lung (*rlung*)
Wind humour

Lungi natsa (*rlung gi na tsha*)
rlung disorder

Lung tsapo (*rlung tsha po*)
Irritability (literally, hot wind), this term is sometimes used in reference to foreigners in Dharamsala

Lung tsogpa (*rlung btsog pa*)
Air pollution

Mani (Sanskrit: *ma ni*)
Avalokiteœvara's mantra *om mani pad me hûm*

Men che ten (*sman dpyad brten*)
Continuing treatment (compliance)

Men drub (*sman grub*)
Empowerment of medicine

Menla (*sman lha*)
Eight Buddhas of medicine

Menla'i do chog (*sman bla'i mdo chog*)
Ritual worship of the Medicine Buddha observed by physicians at the Mentsikhang

Men nga gyu (*sman ngag rgyud*)
The 'Oral Instruction Tantra', the third part of the *Gyushi*

Menpa (*sman pa*)
Traditional Tibetan physician

Menpa kachupa (*sman pa ka chu pa*)
Medical degree given by the Mentsikhang

Mentho (*sman tho*)
Prescription

Mentsikhang (*Sman rtsis khang*)
Tibetan Astro-Medical Institute

Men yanlag gyepa (*sman yan lag brgyad pa*)
The eightfold path of medicine; also refers to the eight branches of medicine: curing, healing, expelling, pharmacology, application of oil, reciting mantras, surgery, and regeneration.

Metsa (*me btsa'*)
Moxibustion

Mi chenpo (*mi chen po*)
Literally a 'big person', an important man or woman

Momo (*mog mog*)
Tibetan dumplings

Monlam (*smon lam*)
Annual prayer festival

Mopa (*mo pa*)
Diviners

Mosar (*mo gsar*)
A virgin (female); short for *bu mo gsar pa*, or literally 'new girl'

Nagpa (*sngags pa*)
Tibetan tantric specialists

Namgyalma (*rnam rgyal ma*)
The all-victorious (Tara) Vijaya, a goddess with three faces and eight arms, Ushnisha-Vijaya

Namshi tangmo (*gnam gshis grang mo*)
Cold weather

Nangmi (*nang mi*)
Close relatives, generally co-residents

Nangmi/kimtse go ne gyabpa (*nang mi/khyim mtshes 'go nad rgyab pa*)
Contagion from family/neighbours

Nata tung (*sna thag 'thung*)
Taking snuff powder

Ngel (*mngal*)
Womb

Ngo (*sngo*)
Herbs

Ngulgi nyogta semtel (*dngul gyi rnyog gra/ sems khral*)
Money problems or worries

Ngulkang yagpo (*dngul khang yag po*)
The 'good bank'

No (*rno*)
Sharp (taste)

Nopa (*gnod pa*)
Harm

Nordag (*nor bdag*)
A wealthy person

Nyam ti (*nyams khrid*)
Teaching through personal experience

Nyam tog (*nyams rtogs*)
Experience (work experience in the context of medical training)

Nyepa (*nyes pa*)
Humour

Nyingi natsa (*snying gi na tsha*)
Heart disorder

Nyingje chenpo (*snying rje chen po*)
Great compassion

Nyingje mena (*snying rje med na*)
Lacking compassion

Nying lung (*snying rlung*)
Heart–*rlung* imbalance

Nying ne (*rnying nad*)
'Old diseases': in the context of Dharamsala's Mentsikhang's education, diseases that are no longer seen in the context of clinical practice

Nying thrag (*rnying khrag*)
Old blood

Oma (*'o ma*)
Milk

Partsa ama (*'phar rtsa a ma*)
Mother vein

Powa'i natsa (*pho ba'i na tsha*)
Stomach disorders

Punkya (*spun kyag*)
Relatives

Rig thun nupa (*rigs mthun nus pa*)
The potency of a medical compound with extracts that come from the same part of the body as the disease which it seeks to cure

Rilbu (*ril bu*)
Precious pill

Rogpa (*'grogs pa*)
Help, companionship

Roma (*ro ma*)
The right channel

Rulwa (*rul ba*)
To rot

Sacha dang namshi gyur (*sa cha dang gnam gshis gyur*)
Changing places and climate

Sacha tangmo dang she tsen (*sa cha grang mo dang bzha' tshan*)
Damp and cold places

Sacha tsawa ne silwar gyur (*sa cha tsha ba nas bsil bar gyur*)
Changing from a hot to a cool place

Samseou (*bsam bse'u*)
Gonads, or organs associated with reproduction

Sang sur (*bsang gsur*)
Incense burning

Sater (*sa gter*)
Minerals

Sem (*sems*)
Mind

Sem gewa (*sems dge ba*)
A virtuous mind (engaged in religious activities)

Sem gyopo (*sems skyo po*)
Having a 'sad mind', feeling depressed

Semtel chepa (*sems khral byed pa*)
To worry

Ser kab (*gser khab*)
Golden needle

Shedang (*zhe sdang*)
Hatred

She gyu (*Bshad rgyud*)
The Explanatory Tantra (the *Gyushi*'s second tantra)

Shelug rolgyur (*zas lugs srol gyur*)
Changing one's food habits

Sherma (*gsher ma*)
Pancreas

Shetsang tsopa / nyogta (*bza' tsang rtsod pa / rnyog khra*)
Marital problems

'shib shib so go re' (*zhib zhib bzos dgos red*)
'You have to powder the medicine.'

Sho (*zho*)
Curd (yogurt)

Shugpa (*shug pa*)
Juniper

Sin (*srin*)
A microorganism, parasite, but also a demon in classical Tibetan

So (*gsos*)
To heal

Sog (*srog*)
Life force

Sokai ne (*gso dka'i nad*)
An illness that is difficult to heal

Sugpo (*gzugs po*)
Body

Sungdue (*srung mdud*)
Protective knot, referring to a knotted string that is blessed and tied to the body

Sungwa (*srung ba*)
Protective charm

Tama tenpa (*tha mag 'then pa*)
Smoking

Tangwa dang tsawa la sogpa'i dugnyel (*grang ba dang tsha ba la sogs pa'i sdug bsngal*)
Hot and cold disorders and similar problems

TB natsa (*Tibi na tsha*)
Tuberculosis

TB nepa nyamdu de (*TB nad pa mnyam du sdod*)
To stay with TB patients

TB sin bu (*Ti bi srin 'bu*)
Microorganisms that cause TB

Teng mo (*phreng mo*)
Divination using prayer beads

Tengwa (*phreng ba*)
Prayer beads

Terma (*gter ma*)
Hidden teaching

Timug (*gti mug*)
Ignorance, stupidity

Tiwa (*dri ba*)
Questioning (in general and as part of a medical consultation)

Tragshe (*khrag shed*)
Blood pressure (also 'high blood pressure', or *khrag shed mtho po*)

Tri dang (*mkhris grang*)
Cold mkhris pa, also used to refer to hepatitis

Tripa'i natsa (*mkhris pa'i na tsha*)
mkhris pa disorder

Tsa (*rtsa*)
Subtle channels, all channels including nerves, veins, arteries, and subtle channels; also used to refer to the 'pulse' of a patient

Tsa gyu (*Rtsa rgyud*)
Root Tantra (first tantra of the *Gyushi*)

Tsa len chig (*rtsa lan gcig*)
One beat of the pulse

Tsa men (*rtswa sman*)
Herbal medicine

Tsa tig (*rtsa thig*)
Channels

Tsawa chi (*tsha ba spyi*)
High fever

Tsawa sum (*rtsa ba gsum*)
The 'three roots' of medicine: aetiology, diagnosis, and therapeutics

Tsetsul ma nyom, tsetsul ma kyi (*tshe tsul ma snyoms, Tshe tsul ma skyid*)
Unbalanced activity levels, unhappy life

Tsigkang (*tshig rkang*)
Versification

Tsipa (*rtsis pa*)
Astrologer

Tso Pema (*Mtsho pad ma*)
Popular pilgrimage destination in Rewalsar (north India); the site is said to be the birthplace of Guru Rinpoche.

Tsog (*tshogs*)
Offerings

Tsuglakang (*Gtsug lag khang*)
Main temple

Tumbu'i natsa (*grum bu'i na tsha*)
Rheumatism, arthritis

Ulpo, dugcha de (*dbul po, sdug cha sdod*)
Living in poor, bad conditions

Uma (*dbu ma*)
The central channel

Wang (*dbang*)
Empowerment; power

Yak (*g.yag*)
Yak

Yiga chupa (*yi ga 'chus pa*)
Repulsion felt while swallowing food, anorexia

Yig tse (*yig tshad*)
Examination

Yul gyarwa (*yul gyar ba*)
Exile, literally someone who has 'changed' location

Zurlug (*zur lugs*)
The 'Zurlug' or southern school of medicine was founded by *Zur mkhar nNyam nyid rDo rje* in the fifteenth century and is one of the two main schools of Tibetan medicine. The other school is commonly known as 'Janglug' (*byang lugs*), or the northern tradition. Gerke (1999) argues that the beginning of the Janglug can be placed roughly half a century earlier than the Zurlug.

Key historical figures and places

Songtsen Gampo
Srong bstan gam po
A Tibetan sovereign who ruled between 629 and 649, according to Shakabpa (1967: 24). The first of the three sovereigns who secured the pre-eminence of Buddhism in Tibet (known as the 'Dharma' kings), Songtsen is credited with consolidating the Yarlung Tibetan state. Songtsen took a Nepalese and a Chinese wife, starting a period of cultural exchange between the three countries. He is said to have invited physicians from India, China, and Persia to Tibet.

Trisong Detsen
Khri srong lde'u btsan
(Ruled *ca.* 754–97) One of the three Dharma kings, Detsen is said to have invited several great physicians from India, Persia, China, and India for a medical conference at Samye (*Bsam yas*) monastery.

Yuthog Yontan Gonpo the Elder
G.yu thog yon tan mgon po Rnying ma
Yuthog the Elder was a personal physician to Trisong Detsen and is said to have visited India several times to receive teachings from Indian physicians. For a full account of Yuthog the Elder's life, see Lobsang Choedak's edition of *Rnam thar bka' rgya ma gzhi brjid rin po che'i gter mdzod*, and his biography in Rechung Rinpoche (1973: 202).

Yuthog Yontan Gonpo the Younger
G.yu thog yon tan mgon po Gsar ma
(*ca.* 1112–1203)
Physician who is said to have compiled, edited, and revised the works composing the *Gyushi*.

Rinchen Sangpo
Rin chen bzang po
(*ca.* 958–1055)
Tibetan scholar and translator whose name is linked to the medical traditional of Tholing (*Mtho lding*) monastery in Western Tibet.

Zurkar Lodoe Gyalpo
Zur mkhar blo gros rgyal po
(*ca.* 1509–79)
The main representative of the 'Zur' school and author of the medical commentary 'Oral Instruction to the Ancestor' (*Mes po'i zhal lung*). Lodoe Gyalpo believed that Yuthog the Younger was the author of the *Gyushi*.

Desi Sangye Gyatso
Sde srid sangs rgyas rgya mthso
(*ca.* 1653–1703/5)
A regent of the 5th Dalai Lama (1617–82), Desi Sangye Gyatso is thought to have synthesised the teachings of the Northern and 'Zur' schools of medicine, as well as founded new medical institutions, including the medical college on the Chagpori hill. The Desi also composed the most influential commentary on the *Gyushi*, the *Blue Beryl* (commonly referred to as *Baidurya sngon po*) He also oversaw the creation of seventy medical *thangkas* illustrating the *Gyushi*.

Drepung monastery
'Bras spungs dgon pa
Founded in 1416 by *'Jam dyangs chos rje bkra shis dpal ldan*, a disciple of *Tsong kha pa*, the fifteenth-century founder of the *dge lugs pa* tradition.

Ganden Phodrang
Dga' ldan pho brang
Lhasa government

Kyenrab Norbu
Mkhyen rab nor bu
(*ca.* 1883–1962)
A prominent director of the Lhasa Mentsikhang, Norbu published numerous textbooks of Tibetan medicine, including a topical outline of the *Rtsa rgyud* and *Bshad rgyud* called *Dpal ldan rtsa ba'i rgyud kyi sdong 'grems gso rig rgya mtsho'i snying po dang bshad rgyud kyi sdoms tshig rgyas bshad sdong 'grems su bkod pa zla shel nor bu'i me long.*

Langdarma
Glang dar ma
Tibetan king who is thought to have ascended to the throne following the death of his brother Ralpacan in 839. Accounts drawing on myth and historical sources report that Langdarma was assassinated by a Buddhist monk in 842. He is widely acknowledged as having played a critical role in the destruction of the heritage of the Tibetan Dharma kings.

Bibliography

Adams, V. 1998. 'Suffering the Winds of Lhasa: Politicized Bodies, Human Rights, Cultural Difference, and Humanism in Tibet'. *Medical Anthropology Quarterly*, 12(1), 74–102.

—. 2001. 'Particularizing Modernity: Tibetan Medical Theorizing of Women's Health in Lhasa, Tibet', in L. Connor and G. Samuel (eds), *Healing Powers and Modernity: Traditional Medicine, Shamanism and Science in Asian Societies*. Westport, CT: Bergin and Garvey, pp. 222–46.

—. 2002a. 'The Sacred in the Scientific: Ambiguous Practices of Science in Tibetan Medicine', *Cultural Anthropology*, 16(4), 542–75.

—. 2002b. 'Establishing Proof: Translating "Science" and the State in Tibetan Medicine', in M. Lock and M. Nichter (eds), *New Horizons in Medical Anthropology: Essays in Honour of Charles Leslie*, London: Bergin and Garvey, pp. 200–20.

—. 2002c. 'Randomized Controlled Crime: Postcolonial Sciences in Alternative Medicine Research', *Social Studies of Science*, 32(5–6), 659–90.

—. 2004. 'Equity of the Ineffable: Cultural and Political Constraints on Ethnomedicine as a Health Problem in Contemporary Tibet' in S.Anand, A. Sen and F. Peter (eds) *Public Health, Ethics, and Equity*. Oxford: Oxford University Press, pp. 283–307.

Adams, V., Miller, S., Craig, S., Sonam, M., Droyoun, L., and Varner, M. 2005. 'The Challenges of Cross-Cultural Clinical Trial Research: A Case Report from the Tibetan Autonomous Region, People's Republic of China', *Medical Anthropology Quarterly*, 19 (3), 267–89.

Ahearn, F. et al. 2000. *Psychosocial Wellness of Refugees: Issues in Qualitative and Quantitative Research*. Oxford: Berghahn Books.

Amnesty International. 2005. *Annual Report 2005*. London: Amnesty International.

Anand, D. 2002. 'A Guide to Little Lhasa in India: The Role of the Symbolic Geography of Dharamsala in Constituting Tibetan Diasporic Identity', in P.C. Klieger (ed.), *Tibet, Self, and the Tibetan Diaspora: Voices of Difference*. PIATS 2000: Proceedings of the Ninth Seminar of the International Association for Tibetan Studies, Leiden 2000. Leiden: Brill's Tibetan Studies Library, pp 11–36.

Anand, S., F. Peter and A. Sen. (eds). 2004. *Public Health, Ethics, and Equity*. Oxford: Oxford University Press.

Arakeri, A.V. 1998. *Tibetans in India: the Uprooted People and their Cultural Transplantation*. New Delhi: Reliance Publishing House.

Ardley, J. 2003. 'Learning the Art of Democracy? Continuity and Change in the Tibetan Government in Exile', *Contemporary South Asia*, 12(3), 349–63.

Argenti-Pillen, A. 2003. *Masking Terror: How Women Contain Violence in Southern Sri Lanka*. Philadelphia: Pennsylvania University Press.

Aspinall, P. 2001. 'Operationalising the Collection of Ethnicity Data in Studies of the Sociology of Health and Illness', *Sociology of Health and Illness*, 23(6), 829–62.

Bhatia, S., T. Dranyi and D. Rowley. 2002a. 'A Social and Demographic Study of Tibetan Refugees in India', *Social Science and Medicine*, 54(3), 411–22.

—. 2002b. 'Tuberculosis among Tibetan Refugees in India', *Social Science and Medicine*, 54(3), 423–32.

Bourgeois, P. 2002. 'Anthropology and Epidemiology on Drugs: the Challenges of Cross-methodological and Theoretical Dialogue', *International Journal of Drug Policy*, 13, 259–69.

Buffetrille, K. 1997. 'The Great Pilgrimage of A myes rma chen: Written Traditions, Living Realities', in A.W. Macdonald (ed.), *Mandala and Landscape*. New Delhi: D.K. Printworld, pp. 75–132.

Braveman, P.A. et al. 2005. 'Socioeconomic Status in Health Research: One size does not fit all', *Journal of the American Medical Association*, 294(22), 2879–88.

Caldwell, L.C. et al. (ed.). 1990. *What We Know about the Health Transition: the Cultural, Social and Behavioral Determinants of Health*. Canberra: Australian National University Press.

Calkowski, M. 1985. Power, Charisma, and Ritual Curing in a Tibetan Community in India. unpublished PhD thesis, University of British Columbia, Department of Anthropology and Sociology.

—. 1991. 'A Day at the Tibetan Opera: Actualized Performance and Spectacular Discourse', *Americal Ethnologist*, 18 (4), 643–57.

Central Tibetan Administration (CTA). 2000. *Tibetan Demographic Survey: 1998*. Dharamsala: Central Tibetan Administration.

Clark, B. 1995. *The Quintessence Tantras of Tibetan Medicine*. Ithaca, NY: Snow Lion Publications.

Clifford, T. 1989. *The Diamond Healing: Tibetan Buddhist Medicine and Psychiatry*. Wellingborough, Northants.: Crucible.

Connor, L.T. 2001. 'Healing Powers in Contemporary Asia', in L. Connor and G. Samuel, (eds), *Healing Powers and Modernity: Traditional Medicine, Shamanism and Science in Asian Societies*. Westport, CT: Bergin and Garvey, pp. 3–21.

Crescenzi, A., E. Ketzer, M. Van Ommeren, K. Phuntsok, I. Komproe and J. de Jong. 2002. 'Effect of Political Imprisonment and Trauma History on Tibetan Refugees in India', *Journal of Traumatic Stress*, 15 (5), 369–75.

Daniel, E.V. 1996. *Charred Lullabies: Chapters in an Anthropology of Violence*. Princeton, NJ: Princeton University Press.

Das, B.C. 1902. *A Tibetan English Dictionary*. New Delhi: Paljor Publications.

Das, V., A. Kleinman, M. Lock, M. Ramphele and P. Reynolds. (eds). 2001. *Remaking A World: Violence, Social Suffering and Recovery*. Berkeley: University of California Press.

Dash, B. 1986. *Tibetan Medicine, With Reference to Yoga Sataka*, 2nd edition. Dharamsala: Library of Tibetan Works and Archives.

De Voe, M.D. 1981. 'Framing Refugees as Clients', *International Migration Review*, 15 (1/2), 88–94.

—. 1983. *Survival of a Refugee Culture: The Longterm Gift Exchange between Tibetan Refugees and Donors in India*. Berkeley: University of California.

Diehl, K. 1997. 'When Tibetan Refugees Rock, Paradigms Roll', in F.J. Korom (ed.), *Constructing Tibetan Culture, Contemporary Perspectives*. St Hyacinthe, Quebec: World Heritage Press, pp. 122–59.

—.2002. *Echoes from Dharamsala: Music in the Life of a Tibetan Refugee Community*. Berkeley: California University Press.

Dorjee, P. 1984. 'Tibetan Medical Treatment of Diabetes, a Case Study', *Tibetan Review*, 19(2), 14–15.

Dreyfus, G. 1999. *The Shugden Affair: Origins of a Controversy*. Dharamsala: CTA, Department of International Relations.

Emmerick, R.E. 1977. 'Sources of the rGyud bzhi', (Supplement, Deuscher Orientalistentag vom 28 Sept. bis Okt. 1975 in Freiburg i. Br.), *Zeitschrift der Deutschen Morgenländischen Gesellschaft*, (Wiesbaden), III (2), 1135–42.

Fadiman, A. 1997. *The Spirit Catches You and You Fall Down*. New York: Farrar, Straus & Giroux.

Farmer, P. 1993. *AIDS and Accusation: Haiti and the Geography of Blame*. Berkeley: University of California Press.

—. 1999. *Infections and Inequalities: The Modern Plagues*. Berkeley: University of California Press.

—. 2003. *Pathologies of Power: Health, Human Rights, and the New War on the Poor*. Berkeley: University of California Press.

Freidson, E. 1970. *Profession of Medicine: A Study of the Sociology of Applied Knowledge*. New York: Dodd, Mead & Company.

Fürer-Haimendorf, C. 1990. *The Renaissance of the Tibetan Civilization*. London: Synergetic Press.

Gardner, K. 2002. *Age, Narrative and Migration: The Life Course and Life Histories of Bengali Elders in London*. London: Berg.

Gerke, B. 1998. 'Problems of Translating and Creating Tibetan Medical Terminology', unpublished paper presented at the First International Conference on Tibetan Medicine, Washington DC, 7–9 November 1998. Available from the author.

—. 1999. 'On the History of the Two Tibetan Medical Schools Janglug and Zurlug', AyurVijnana, 5. Available online: http://www.ittm.org/publications/AyurVijnana/ Vol_06/AV_V06_3.htm (accessed 24 July 2007).

—. 2001. 'Die Problematik der Tibetischen Medizin im Kontakt mit dem Westen', unpublished paper presented at the Institut fur Allgemeinmedizin, Klinikum der Johann Wolfgang Goethe Universitat, Frankfurt am Main, 24 April 2001. Available from the author.

Graham H. 2002. 'Building an Inter-disciplinary Science of Health Inequalities: The Example of Life Course Research', *Social Science and Medicine*, 55, 2005–16.

Grove, N.J. and A.B. Zwi. 2005. 'Our Health and Theirs: Forced Migration, Othering, and Public Health', *Social Science and Medicine*, 62(8), 1931–42.

Harris, C. 1999. *In the Image of Tibet: Tibetan Painting after 1959*. London: Reaktion Books.

Holtz, T. 1998. 'Refugee Trauma versus Torture Trauma: A Retrospective Controlled Cohort Study of Tibetan Refugees', *Journal of Nervous and Mental Disease*, 186(1), 24–34.

Huber, T. 1999. 'Book Review [online] of Korom, F.J., (ed.), Constructing Tibetan Culture: Contemporary Perspectives', *Journal of Buddhist Ethics* [online]. Available from: http://jbe.gold.ac.uk/5/huber981.htm).

Janes, C.R. 1995. 'The Transformations of Tibetan Medicine', *Medical Anthropology Quarterly*, 9, 6–39.

—. 2001. 'Tibetan Medicine at the Crossroads: Radical Modernity and the Social Organization of Traditional Medicine in the Tibet Autonomous Region, China', in L. Connor and G. Samuel (eds), *Healing Powers and Modernity: Traditional Medicine, Shamanism and Science in Asian Societies*. Westport, CT: Bergin and Garvey, pp. 197–222.

Karmay, S.G. 1989. 'Vairocana and the rGyud bzhi', *Tibetan Medicine*, 12, 19–31.

Klieger, P.C. 2002. *Tibet, Self, and the Tibetan Diaspora: Voices of Difference*. PIATS 2000: Proceedings of the Ninth Seminar of the International Association for Tibetan Studies, Leiden 2000. Leiden: Brill's Tibetan Studies Library.

Leslie, C. 1976. *Asian Medical Systems: A Comparative Study*. Berkeley, Los Angeles and London: University of California Press.

Lopez, D.S. 1998. *Prisoners of Shangri La: Tibetan Buddhism and the West*. Chicago: University of Chicago Press.

McKay, A. 2005. 'The Birth of a Clinic? The IMS Dispensary in Gyantse (Tibet) 1904–1910', *Medical History*, 49(2), 135–54.

McKay, L., S. Mcintyre and A. Ellaway. 2003. *Migration and Health: A Review of the International Literature*. MRC Social and Public Health Sciences Unit, Occasional Paper No. 12: www.msoc-mrc.gla.ac.uk/Publications/pub/PDFs/Occasional-Papers/OP012-Text.pdf (accessed 20 July 2007).

Malkki, L. 1992. 'National Geographic: The Rooting of Peoples and the Territorialization of National Identity among Scholars and Refugees', *Cultural Anthropology*, 7(1), 24–44.

—. 1995a. *Purity and Exile: Violence, Memory, and National Cosmology among Hutu Refugees in Tanzania*. Chicago: University of Chicago Press.

—. 1995b. 'Refugees and Exile: From "Refugee Studies" to the National Order of Things', *Annual Review of Anthropology*, 24, 495–523.

Marmot, M. 2004. *Status Syndrome: How Our Position on the Social Gradient Affects Longevity and Health*. London and New York: Bloomsbury Publishing.

Mentsikhang. 1995. *Fundamentals of Tibetan Medicine according to the Gyushi*. Dharamsala: Mentsikhang (Tibetan Medical and Astrological Institute of His Holiness the Dalai Lama).

—. 1998. *Proceedings of the Conference on Clinical Research in Tibetan Medicine: Panel Discussions, Lectures and Papers*. Dharamsala: Mentsikhang.

Mercer, S., A. Ager and E. Ruwanpura. 2005. 'Psychosocial Distress of Tibetan Exiles: Integrating Western Interventions with Traditional Beliefs and Practices', *Social Science and Medicine*, 60(1), 179–89.

Meyer, F. 1992. 'Introduction', in Y. Parfionovitch, F. Meyer and G. Dorje. (eds), *Tibetan Medical Paintings: Illustration of the Blue Beryl Treatise of Sangye Gyamtso (1653–1705)*. London: Serindia.

—. 2002. *gSo ba Rig pa, Le Système médical tibétain*. Paris: Editions du Centre national de la Recherche Scientifique.

Millard, C. 2002. Learning Processes in a Tibetan Medical School, unpublished thesis, University of Edinburgh, Department of Social Anthropology.

Mishra, P. 2000. *The Romantics*. London: Anchor Books.

Morrissey, J. 1983. 'Migration, Resettlement, and Refugeeism: Issues in Medical Anthropology', *Medical Anthropology Quarterly*, 15(1), 11–14.

Moynihan, M. 1997. *Tibetan Refugees in India and Nepal*. Testimony before the Senate Foreign Relations Committee Hearing on Tibet on 13 May 1997 [online]. Available from: http://www.tibet.ca/wtnarchive/1997/5/20_3.html.

Namdul, T., A. Sood, L. Ramakrishnan, R.M. Pandey and D. Moorthy. 2001. 'Efficacy of Tibetan Medicine as an Adjunct in the Treatment of Type 2 Diabetes', *Diabetes Care*, 24(1), 175–77.

Nazroo, J.Y. 2001. *Ethnicity, Class and Health*. London: Policy Studies Institute.

Nelson, L.J., Y. Naik, K. Tsering and J.P. Cegielski. 2005. 'Population-based Risk Factors for Tuberculosis and Adverse Outcomes among Tibetan Refugees in India, 1994–1996', *International Journal of Tuberculosis and Lung Disease*, 9(9), 1018–26.

Nguyen, V.K. and K. Peschard. 2003. 'Anthropology, Inequality and Disease: A Review', *Annual Review of Anthropology*, 32, 447–74.

Nichter, M. 1989. 'Idioms of Distress, Alternatives in the Expression of Psychosocial Distress: A Case Study from South India', *Culture, Medicine and Psychiatry*, 5, 379–408.

Norbu, J. 1998. Interview [online]. In Dreams of Tibet, Frontline. Available from: http://www.pbs.org/wgbh/pages/frontline/shows/tibet/interviews/norbu.html

Ong, A. 1999. *Flexible Citizenship: the Cultural Logics of Transnationality*. Durham, NC: Duke University Press.

Palakshappa, T.C. 1978. *Tibetans in India: A Case Study of Mundgod Tibetan*. New Delhi: Sterling Publishers.

Parfionovitch, Y., G. Dorje and F. Meyer. 1992. *Tibetan Medical Paintings: Illustration of the Blue Beryl Treatise of Sangye Gyamtso (1653–1705)*. London: Serindia.

Parry, J.P. 1979. *Caste and Kinship in Kangra*. London, Henley & Boston: Routledge & Kegan Paul.

Pearce N. and D.G. Smith. 2003. 'Is Social Capital the Key to Inequalities in Health?' *American Journal of Public Health*, 93(1), 122–29.

Prost, A. 2004. 'Infectious Social Change: Tuberculosis and Exile among Tibetan Refugees in Dharamsala', in M. Worton and N. Wilson-Tagoe (eds), *National Healths: Gender, Sexuality and Health in a Cross-cultural Context*. London: UCL Press, pp. 170–78.

—. 2006a. 'Causation as Strategy: Interpreting Humours among Tibetan Refugees', *Anthropology and Medicine*, 13(2), 119–30.

—. 2006b. The Problem with 'Rich Refugees': Sponsorship, Capital, and the Informal Economy of Tibetan Refugees, *Modern Asian Studies*, 40(1), 233–54.

Punkhill, D. 1992. *Tibetan Health, the First Decade 1981–1991*. Report from Dharamsala: Department of Health, Central Tibetan Administration.

Rabgay, L. 1994a. 'Pulse Analysis in Tibetan Medicine', *Tibetan Medicine*, 3, 47–54.

—. 1994b. 'Urine Analysis in Tibetan Medicine', *Tibetan Medicine*, 3, 55–62.

Ramble, C. and K. Buffetrille (eds). 1998. *Tibétains. 1959–1999: 40 Ans de Colonisation*. Paris: éditions Autrement, collection Monde HS, no. 108.

Saklani, G. 1984. *The Uprooted Tibetans in India: a Sociological Study of Community and Change*. Delhi: Cosmo Publications.

Samuel, G. 1993. *Civilized Shamans: Buddhism in Tibetan Societies*. Washington and London: Smithsonian Institution Press.

—. 2001. 'Tibetan Medicine in Contemporary India: Theory and Practice', in L. Connor and G. Samuel (eds), *Healing Powers and Modernity: Traditional Medicine, Shamanism and Science in Asian Societies*. Westport, CT: Bergin and Garvey, pp. 247–67.

Samten [Bsam gtan]. 1997. The New Dawn Condensed Compendium of Healing Knowledge [*Gso rig snying bsdus skya rengs gsar pa*]. Lhasa: Tibet People's Publishing House [*Bod ljongs ni dmangs dpe skrun khang*].

Scheper-Hughes, N. and M. Lock. 1987. 'The Mindful Body: A Prolegomenon to Future Work in Medical Anthropology'. *Medical Anthropology Quarterly*, 1(1), 6–41.

Schrempf, M. and F. Garret. 2003. 'What is Bon Medicine? Analysing Narratives of Illness and Healing in the History and Practice of a Lesser Known Tibetan Medical Tradition', *IIAS Newsletter*, 30, International Institute for Asian Studies, Leiden, S. 29.

Seidman, S. 1997. *Aids in India and its Potential Impact on the Tibetan Refugee Community* [online]. Available from: http://itsa.ucsf.edu/~seidman/taids10.html.

Shakabpa, W.D. 1967. *Tibet: A Political History*. New Haven: Yale University Press.

Shakya, T. 1999. *The Dragon in the Land of Snows*. London: Pimlico.

Sinclair, S. 1997. *Making Doctors: An Institutional Apprenticeship*. Oxford: Berg.

Sontag, S. 1978. *Illness as Metaphor, AIDS and its Metaphors*. London: Penguin Books.

Stein, R.A. 1972. *Tibetan Civilization*. Stanford: Stanford University Press.

Subba, T.B. 1990. *Flight and Adaptation: Tibetan Refugees in the Darjeeling-Sikkim Himalaya*. Dharamsala: Library of Tibetan Works and Archives.

Tibet Information Network. 2002. *Delivery and Deficiency: Health and Health Care in Tibet* [report]. London: TIN.

Trostle, J. 2005. *Epidemiology and Culture*. Cambridge and New York: Cambridge University Press.

Trostle, J. and J. Sommerfeld. 1996. 'Medical Anthropology and Epidemiology', *Annual Review of Anthropology*, 25, 253–74.

Tsundue, T. 2005. *My Tibetanness*. [poem] Available on: http://www.tibetwrites.org/ poems/tt.html (accessed 24 July 2007).

Wares, D.F., T.D. Sadutshang, N.J. Beeching and P. Davies. 2000. 'Control of Tuberculosis amongst the Tibetan Refugee Community in Northern India', *Indian Journal of Tuberculosis*, 47, 35–41.

Wilkinson, R.G. 1996. *Unhealthy Societies: The Afflictions of Inequality*. London: Routledge.

Wylie, T. 1959. 'A Standard System of Tibetan Transcription', *Harvard Journal of Asiatic Studies*, 22, 261–67.

Index

www.ingramcontent.com/pod-product-compliance
Ingram Content Group UK Ltd.
Pitfield, Milton Keynes, MK11 3LW, UK
UKHW021833100926
8556IPUK00004B/318

9 781845 454579